Praise for *Daring to*

"As someone who has found yoga nidra to be utterly life changing, I am over-the-moon delighted that Karen wrote a guide for every woman to get the rest she needs using this ancient tool. You'll love the science and the excellent case she makes for why you need rest. But the way she gives you to actually get that rest—it's going to create such magic in your life. Please read this and *do* the practices. Then prepare to become a raving fan!"

> **JENNIFER LOUDEN**
> author of *The Woman's Comfort Book* and *The Life Organizer*

"What a masterpiece! With skill and compassion, Karen masterfully guides her reader through a step-by-step journey into herself, where she can shed the worn-out woman and emerge well rested, fully energized, and empowered. Accessible, relatable, and full of inspirational success stories, this book artfully introduces the ancient practice of yoga nidra rest meditation to our rest-deprived society."

> **KAMINI DESAI, PHD**
> author of *Yoga Nidra: The Art of Transformational Sleep*,
> education director of Amrit Yoga Institute

"Karen Brody's *Daring to Rest* offers us essential teachings about the true nature and profound benefits of genuine rest . . . Based on an integration of science and spirituality, Karen gently guides us through an effective and practical, life-changing program . . . *Daring to Rest* is a beautiful book of contagious inspiration."

> **RUBIN NAIMAN, PHD**
> clinical assistant professor of medicine,
> University of Arizona Center for Integrative Medicine

"*Daring to Rest* is simply brilliant. I thought I knew a thing or two about health, rest, and yoga. But in this wonderful book, Karen Brody breathes new life into the need for rest—and it's not just 'get more sleep.' After reading *Daring to Rest*, I cannot *wait* to lie down, listen to a yoga nidra meditation, and start listening to my soul. Women everywhere need to take rest seriously if they are to enjoy vibrant health. This book is the most practical place to start."

CHRISTIANE NORTHRUP, MD
OB/GYN physician and author of the *New York Times*
bestsellers *Goddesses Never Age; Women's Bodies,*
Women's Wisdom; and *The Wisdom of Menopause*

"In this world that tells us that in order to be more we must keep doing more and more, *Daring to Rest* is a beautiful, true antidote. The truth is that the only way to have what we really want is to stop, rest, and make space. *Daring to Rest* is the perfect guide to do just that. Read this book, follow this wisdom, and enjoy the experience of truthful living that can only come from a well-rested place."

KATE NORTHRUP
bestselling author of *Money: A Love Story*

"In *Daring to Rest*, Karen Brody skillfully shows us how to discover deep, restorative rest and maintain core relaxation amidst the challenges we all face in our daily lives. Karen's true gift is her ability to showcase ancient meditative principles in simple, secular practices that restore and support health and well-being at all levels of our body and mind. Karen expertly guides us—in easy-to-follow steps—in how to interweave these elegant, simple, yet profound practices into our daily life."

RICHARD MILLER, PHD
author of *iRest Meditation, The iRest Program*
for Healing PTSD, and *Yoga Nidra: A Meditative*
Practice for Deep Relaxation and Healing

"As a mindfulness teacher, I know how meditation creates such rest through synchronizing mind and body. Yoga nidra provides the same pathway to this calm, well-rested place where power and purpose are rediscovered. Karen's new book brings together rest, meditation, and women's empowerment to create lasting benefits when it comes to sleep, mood, and overall happiness."

SUSAN PIVER
author of *Start Here Now: An Open-Hearted*
Guide to the Path and Practice of Meditation

"Karen Brody has put together a program that makes yoga nidra relevant and accessible to 21st-century women, who may need the practice more than any previous generation. If you feel overwhelmed by living, the techniques in *Daring to Rest* are a good place to start your journey back to well-being."

SHARON SALZBERG
author of *Lovingkindness* and *Real Love*

"*Daring to Rest* is a book that every woman can benefit from. . . . Karen shares a journey of 40 days to rest and rise, which to me is the garden of life many women are searching for . . . I highly recommend this beautiful piece of art."

KARENA VIRGINIA
healer, speaker, TV personality, and author
of *Essential Kundalini Yoga*

"In this over-committed, gadget-obsessed world, most of us have forgotten what true rest feels like. *Daring to Rest* is a much-needed clarion call that reminds us how to find freedom in a restful body, mind, and spirit. Karen Brody's authentic voice and her elegant 40-day program will bring you home, at last, to rest, release, and rise."

JEFFREY DAVIS
author, speaker, and creativity consultant

DARING
TO REST

KAREN BRODY

DARING TO REST

Reclaim Your Power with
Yoga Nidra Rest Meditation

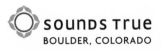

SOUNDS TRUE
BOULDER, COLORADO

Sounds True
Boulder, CO 80306

Published 2017

This book is not intended as a substitute for the medical recommendations of
physicians, mental health professionals, or other health-care providers. Rather, it is
intended to offer information to help the reader cooperate with physicians, mental
health professionals, and health-care providers in a mutual quest for optimal well-
being. We advise readers to carefully review and understand the ideas presented
and to seek the advice of a qualified professional before attempting to use them.

Some names and identifying details have been changed to protect the privacy
of individuals.

Cover design by Jennifer Miles
Book design by Beth Skelley

Cover image © Golubvoy, shutterstock.com

Printed in Canada

Library of Congress Cataloging-in-Publication Data
Names: Brody, Karen, author.
Title: Daring to rest : reclaim your power with Yoga Nidra rest meditation /
   Karen Brody.
Description: Boulder, CO : Sounds True, 2017. | Includes bibliographical references.
Identifiers: LCCN 2017010827 (print) | LCCN 2017011784 (ebook) |
   ISBN 9781622039104 (ebook) | ISBN 9781622039098 (pbk.)
Subjects: LCSH: Hatha yoga. | Relaxation. | Meditation.
Classification: LCC RA781.7 (ebook) | LCC RA781.7 .B7574 2017 (print) |
   DDC 613.7/046—dc23
LC record available at https://lccn.loc.gov/2017010827

10 9 8 7 6 5 4 3 2 1

For R., women, and humanity.

If you close your eyes,
you will see far.

KENYAN PROVERB

CONTENTS

CONTENTS

DEAR SISTER,

Welcome. I wrote this book for you as an invitation to improve your well-being and dream big using *yoga nidra*, a meditative practice that can help you realize true, deep rest. Through these pages, you can discover your path back to whatever your heart desires, including better sleep, clarity of mind, loving relationships, and the courage to make a difference in the world. I wrote this book to help women get some much-needed rest, reclaim their radiant nature, and lead at home and work from a more peaceful place. I felt called to share with you a meditation technique that is both practical and life changing and that will help you give birth to *anything* in your life from a well-rested place.

I could speak for days and months and years about yoga nidra meditation. Why? Because yoga nidra transformed my life, and I have seen it, again and again, in some way, change the life of every woman it touches. Yoga nidra combines what I feel are two key components women need in their lives: a well-rested body and a deep connection to one's soul. A well-rested, healthy body helps the soul fulfill its purpose.

This book shows you how to make peace an inside job. I am convinced that if more women (and men) practiced yoga nidra, we would create a more peaceful world because we would all be more at peace with ourselves. We would all sleep better. We would prioritize being good to ourselves. We would stop chronically burning out, and if we did burn out, we would quickly forgive ourselves, chuck "perfect," and reboot. We would bravely tell the untold stories wanting out of our heads and finally release story lines that no longer serve us. We would lead more companies and feel more confident and creative, doing it *our* way instead of how it's always been done (which isn't working for women, by the way). We would model to our children how to not be afraid of the dark—within us or outside of us.

My first yoga nidra teacher, Robin Carnes, always ended her yoga nidra meditation sessions with the words, "Yoga nidra is a service of love we give to ourselves and all others. It mentors us into an understanding of our true nature, and it shows us that when we serve ourselves, we serve all others; when we serve others, we serve ourselves."

This is the spirit from which this book is being offered to you. May this book help you be good to yourself, rest well, heal, lead, be wildly creative, and stand in your full power. May it also help you recover a deep sense of peace within and then go spread peace to others.

The time is now to take back rest.

Let's do this—together.

With love and shaking my yoga nidra pompoms,
Karen

INTRODUCTION

Fifteen years ago, I was a young mom with two active boys under the age of two. My older son slept so little and cried so much that for over a year we ate every meal with the vacuum cleaner on just to keep him calm. Living with so much tension and so little sleep made me feel and act *crazypants*. My everyday thoughts included things like, "What day is it?" and "Oh, was that a curb I just drove over?"

I had been a confident young woman, and I had lots of experience as a leader. But once sleep deprivation and chronic stress hit, my confidence sank to an all-time low. "Who am I again?" and "All I want to do is sleep" became my mantras. That's when a family legacy of panic attacks kicked in unexpectedly, in my local supermarket, and I began taking anti-anxiety pills.

"I'm *fine*," I told everyone. It made sense that I would be constantly exhausted and full of panic. For a mom in this situation, there was no other way to be, right?

Turns out I was wrong. There was another way.

I found it by accident when I wandered into my local yoga studio. As I read through the class choices, I heard a voice echoing in the hallway. Attracted to its energy, I walked toward the voice and found twenty or so women lying on the floor with blankets over them, looking blissed out. The woman at the front desk told me it was a yoga nidra class.

"What are they doing?" I asked her.

"I guess you could say they're doing nothing. It's like taking a yogic nap."

She explained that yoga nidra is "the art of conscious relaxation" and said it is also known as "the sleep of the yogi." I was already familiar with meditation, though I hadn't meditated in years, and what she described sounded like a kind of meditation, but one I could do lying down instead of sitting up. I signed up for the class immediately.

A week later, I stood at the classroom door, took a deep breath, walked in, and lay down. To be honest, even though I had years of experience in meditation, I wasn't looking to meditate or even "consciously relax." I was just desperate to lie down and get some rest.

What I got was the best rest of my life. It also turned out to be the first step on my journey to feeling like myself again—my truest, most powerful self.

Right away my weekly yoga nidra sessions felt deeply restorative in my physical body. My nervous system was no longer permanently on high alert, and I felt rested for the first time in a long while. But suddenly there was more. As I continued practicing yoga nidra, something began to tug at my core. A portal was opening. At times my heart would flutter, making me wonder, *What is this new thing wanting to emerge?* I was being nudged to take a close look at my "fine" life and make some changes.

At the same time, there was a part of me hollering, "Curl back up to *fine!*" The temptation to not change a thing in my busy life, and to not rest, was looping through my mind most days for a few months or so after I began practicing yoga nidra meditation regularly. I loved it, and yet every Friday at noon, when my yoga nidra class met, I had a long list of excuses to not lie down. Shifting lifelong patterns can be a one-step-forward, one-step-back dance, but over time, the yoga nidra magic kept calling me back, and I gave myself permission to rest more, slow down, and not live in the "fine" zone.

As I began to feel well rested, I tapped back into my own internal rhythm, something I had neglected for a long time. Every time I lay down to practice yoga nidra, I felt the weight of all I was doing, and it became clear that I was stressed. And from a deep, meditative space connected to my natural rhythm, I was led to solutions to my stress. Everything that had felt urgent began to feel less urgent. I began to clear nonessential things from my schedule, and the sense of freedom from my to-do list was intoxicating. I started unplugging from the computer before dinner and didn't go back afterward, so I could focus on my family and myself and then wind down before bedtime and get a good night's sleep. I didn't call friends back during the week—only on weekends, when I could go for a relaxing walk while talking. I said no to anything that made me feel out of rhythm, like unessential family travel or too many weekend activities.

Soon after I made yoga nidra an ongoing priority, my panic attacks disappeared. I realized that my family history did not have to become my reality, and in that first year of practicing yoga nidra meditation, I was able to stop taking anti-anxiety medication. It wasn't easy to stop the medication, but practicing yoga nidra showed me that I could do it—that feeling calm and free was my birthright. Slowly, as I continued practicing yoga nidra, I began to connect back to all the original dreams I'd had as a young girl, like wanting to write. I released a big story I'd been telling myself for years: that a dyslexic who wasn't allowed to take an English class in college couldn't write. During yoga nidra, I kept hearing a whisper from my soul to "screw that story and write a play." So I wrote a successful play called *Birth*, which came straight from my soul. Yoga nidra reminded me that storytelling is in my bones, and if we don't follow the wisdom in our bones, a part of us dies. It also showed me how deep rest and stillness could profoundly improve my health and leadership. I didn't have to spend years as a worn-out woman, thinking this was a badge of honor or just the way you're supposed to feel as a mother. After this, there was no turning back to just "fine."

What About You? Are You Just "Fine"?

If you're a woman in today's high-paced modern world, there's a good chance you feel like I did all those years ago. Maybe, like me, you've been listening to the conventional wisdom for a long time: *All mothers are tired. All women who work are crazy busy. Being tired all the time is normal.* Maybe, like me, you tell yourself and others that you're fine, not realizing that *fine* is often code for "my life isn't going well." It's easy to think worn out is normal because the worn-out woman model is the dominant model for women in our culture. Have you noticed how our culture loves women achievers, even if they're exhausted every step of the way to the top?

Maybe you've tinkered around with empowerment tools and the latest health advice: *Exercise more. Eat leafy greens. Drink more water. Buy supplements. No, you've got to get the "right" supplements. Try probiotics.* While these things often help when combined with rest, on their own, they typically aren't solutions. They're just stopgaps helping a tired body keep going a little more, and you're sucked back into exhaustion again when confronted with the daily demands of life and not enough time.

Maybe, like I was, you're taking some type of medication to help you feel better or sleep better. Maybe you're thinking, "I don't have the time for rest" or "How can rest really make a huge difference?" Maybe you're wondering if daring to rest is worth the risk.

If any of this sounds familiar, I invite you take stock of your life now. Review any current physical, mental, and emotional health issues, including the red flags you may have been ignoring for years, and then ask yourself, "Am I thriving?" Not just living, not just fine, but really *thriving*? Are you really the woman you want to be and that you know you could be, if you were operating at full power? Do you feel healthy? If the answer is no, how could deep, nourishing rest help you thrive? Is it worth the risk?

I wrote *Daring to Rest* and created the Daring to Rest program to help women give up the all-too-familiar worn-out woman paradigm and replace it with an urgently needed, well-rested one. What I'm offering you in this book is a rest program that will help you reboot your health and your life so that you can begin dreaming big and leading from a well-rested place. I will reteach you how to rest deeply and then use this as fuel to live your life from a more peaceful, authentic, and purposeful place.

The world needs you and what you have to offer. But it needs the fully alive, well-rested you, not the exhausted you. Imagine a world where women make rest and rhythm a priority and operate more from their full power. That's the new daring-to-rest world you're about to enter.

Daring to Rest: The Program

After experiencing firsthand the profound changes yoga nidra can lead to, I became an uncharacteristically enthusiastic yoga nidra cheerleader. Years after I started practicing, I realized that yoga nidra made my heart sing, and I sought out training in two different yoga nidra methods. From there, I developed Bold Tranquility, a company dedicated to showing worn-out women their way back to deep rest and their purpose through the benefits of yoga nidra meditation.

This book will lead you through the Daring to Rest program, in which you practice yoga nidra meditation for forty days in order to break the cycle of fatigue, feel healthy again, and reconnect to your soul's calling—the woman you are when you're not completely, constantly exhausted.

The yoga nidra meditations will teach you how to step into a deeply restful, timeless state that relaxes your body and helps you feel physically rested. But physical exhaustion is just the first layer of exhaustion. If it were the only layer, then just getting more sleep or sleeping better would resolve fatigue. Yoga nidra meditation helps you clear the burnout you're experiencing at the deeper, subtler levels of your being so that you can feel rested and whole again on not just the physical body level, but mental, emotional, and spiritual levels as well.

Chapter one explains what real rest is (Hint: It's not just another self-care activity) and why it is so important for modern women. Chapters two and three provide you with everything you need to know about yoga nidra meditation and how the Daring to Rest program works.

Then the second, third, and fourth sections of the book lead you through the forty-day program's three phases:

"Phase One: Rest" addresses physical exhaustion.

"Phase Two: Release" addresses mental and emotional exhaustion.

"Phase Three: Rise" addresses the "life-purpose exhaustion" that typically arises when we are not operating at our full power.

At the end of the Rise phase, I will show you how to incorporate yoga nidra meditation and other principles and practices from this book into your life, so you can continue to make rest a priority—because a well-rested lifestyle is forever.

Please note that while the program is forty days, it takes into account real life and gives you permission to not practice some days—because chucking perfect is a much-needed skill for well-rested women too.

In addition to the yoga nidra meditations themselves, I offer complementary practices in each chapter, from writing to movement to harnessing your power to access intuitive guidance. Women are multidimensional, so often the way into healing varies from woman to woman. Pick and choose what suits you.

Throughout the book, I share some of my stories and the stories of women I've worked with in my programs, hoping they provide you with guidance, assurance, and awareness on your journey. Many of the women's names have been changed, and some stories are composites to capture the essence of the teachings. I'm deeply grateful to every woman who bravely said yes to sharing her story. The protective mama in me asks you to deeply listen, respect their truths, and feel into (or "think with your heart") how they relate to your truth.

Since I'm an enthusiastic yoga nidra cheerleader, I will be shaking my yoga nidra pompoms throughout this book, not just because yoga nidra helped me go from an exhausted, worn-out woman to a more well-rested woman, and not just because I've seen it do the same for other women, but also because I know that on a deep, cellular level, yoga nidra heals many dimensions of ourselves and infuses us with unspeakable courage in all areas of our lives—courage to give ourselves permission to rest, and more. When you lie down with yoga nidra, you are guided into stillness, and it's through discovering this inherent stillness in yourself that you find freedom.

Now, my dear Sister, it's time to lie down and begin the journey to waking up.

THE
FOUNDATION

1

WHY REST IS SO IMPORTANT FOR WOMEN

You probably don't need to be convinced how important it is to rest. You know you're exhausted, stressed out, and frazzled. And you're not alone. Consider these statistics:

- In a 2014 report by the National Sleep Foundation, 24 percent of women said they had woken up feeling well rested for zero of the past seven days.[1]

- Women have more insomnia and higher depression levels than men.[2]

- The number of women aged 20–44 taking medications for attention deficit hyperactivity disorder (ADHD) increased 264 percent between 2001 and 2010.[3]

Do you truly think that the number of women having problems with focus and attention suddenly jumped for no clear reason? Of course not. This dramatic rise in medication use is our cry for help. Add to this the high numbers of women taking medication for depression—in one survey, 23 percent of all American women between the ages of 40 and 59—and one thing is clear: women are out of rhythm.[4] And how do you come back into rhythm? Rest. What if the inexpensive treatment of *rest* could give women their lives back?

Sleep specialist Rubin Naiman, PhD, says, "Buddhist philosophy teaches that depression results from excessive activation that is not properly balanced by rest."[5] By "activation," he means that nonstop doing keeps our sympathetic nervous systems on high alert all the time. This Buddhist take on depression makes sense when I think of many of the women I support: They're very busy and rarely rest. Many are on multiple medications, and most feel significantly better—and quite a few are virtually cured of insomnia, anxiety, and depression—once they consistently practice yoga nidra meditation. You can be busy, and even occasional stress is okay and quite normal, but you must balance it with rest and relaxation—otherwise, it's a recipe for burnout.

What if, instead of putting women on medication or telling us to cure our health issues with a checklist of ten steps, we put them on an intense rest program first and then supported their unique needs as they began to feel whole again? What if rest could teach us the holy grail of womanhood: chucking perfect? And what if resting and restoring flow in our bodies, minds, and spirits is the key to more effective, sustainable women's leadership? This is why I created the Daring to Rest program. I want you to try rest as a remedy. I want you to feel how deep rest can change your life. Now, with this program, any woman can easily plug in to rest for forty days and see how it begins to change her life.

Years ago I interviewed a nutritionist who helps women lose weight. She told me that for a long time, her first step was to get women on specialized diets. But now, before asking them to make any dietary changes, she has them chart their sleep for one month and then work on improving their sleep. Why? Because trying to lose weight when you're sleep deprived is much more challenging than trying to lose weight when you're well rested.

What's clear is that rest is key to well-being and that women's well-being is suffering. In my world, all roads lead back to the importance of deep rest.

What Exactly Is Rest?

When I ask women what their self-care activities are, they often tell me things like this: take a bike ride, read a book, go to the movies, meet a girlfriend for dinner, have a glass of wine, play a game (often on a smartphone). There's nothing wrong with these activities, but they should not be considered rest. Rest is not active. To rest is to surrender from the active, the goals, and the will to achieve something. Activities like going for a bike ride keep you focused on your outer world. Rest invites you to experience the gentle exchange between your outer and inner worlds.

In his book *Consolations*, the poet and essayist David Whyte deliciously captures what rest really is and describes it as having five states:

> **In the first state of rest is the sense of stopping, of giving up on what we have been doing or how we have been being. In the second, is the sense of slowly coming home, the physical journey into the body's un-coerced and un-bullied self. . . . In the third state is a sense of healing and self-forgiveness and of arrival. In the fourth state . . . is the give and the take, the blessing and the being blessed and the ability to delight in both. The fifth stage is a sense of absolute readiness and presence, a delight in and an anticipation of the world and all its forms; a sense of being the meeting itself between inner and outer, and that receiving and responding occur in one spontaneous movement.**[6]

There seems to be a huge number of women who don't know how to rest. My hand is raised here too. I'm a mom, and it took me a while to understand that as much as I enjoyed sitting down to watch a movie at the end of the day, that was recreation, not rest. Activities such as reading a book or knitting are also not rest because while they are physically relaxing, they engage your eyes and mind, keeping you mentally active and alert.

Most self-care today is about activation or doing—exercising, taking a trip with friends, going out to dinner. While this activation may nurture parts of your body, mind, and spirit, it does not deeply replenish your mind and body. Being busy stimulates the sympathetic nervous system, the part of your autonomic nervous system that controls your "fight-or-flight" response. If you live in active, busy mode for long periods of time, keeping only the sympathetic nervous system active, you put stress on your entire nervous system. The result? Anxiety, depression, and sleep disorders. To reduce this stress, you must take time to stimulate the opposite part of the autonomic nervous system—the parasympathetic nervous system—for balance.

Giving yourself nonactive time allows not only your physical body the opportunity to rest and rejuvenate, but also your mind. The key feature of rest that distinguishes it from other forms of self-care is that it invites you to step out of your everyday life and dip into your inner world, the space where wonder and creativity flourish and where you can discover a fresh perspective on your everyday life. Rest could be sitting in a chair at dusk and quietly observing the sunset. You are essentially doing nothing, but by allowing yourself to rest in a gap of nothingness, where your thoughts slow down, you can get out of your mind and, often, touch the mysterious familiarity of your soul. Meditation and some types of yoga can take you to this same gap of nothingness. Sleep and a good nap can do this too. Deep sleep can take us to our inner world. Dream exploration does too.

The result is often feeling as if you have rebooted your entire system because when you rest, you stimulate your parasympathetic nervous system, the "rest-and-digest" function of your overall autonomic nervous system. But many people are not sleeping well or dreaming much, which is why we need rest practices like yoga nidra meditation—to teach us how to enter our internal world.

Why Rest Is the Ideal Remedy for Women Today

Why is deep rest an ideal remedy for worn-out women today? Here are three important reasons.

Rest Is Part of Our Natural Cycles

After you do something active, it is best to follow up with something that is less active. Pioneering sleep researcher Nathaniel Kleitman called this pattern our "basic rest-activity cycle," or BRAC.[7] He observed that our bodies typically operate in ninety-minute cycles, both when we're asleep and awake. As we transition from waking to light sleep, our brain waves slowly lower. A healthy sleeper will transition in the second half of the BRAC period to high brain waves, a deeper sleep stage. This cycle continues every ninety minutes. When we're awake, our brain waves are faster for the first half of the BRAC, and then our brain waves begin to slow down, which is why we often get tired and less focused as we get closer to the end of a ninety-minute period of concentration.[8]

The problem comes when we override this cycle by deciding to not take a break after ninety minutes. This is often when we reach for pseudo-fuel, such as caffeine or sugar, to keep going on high alert for longer than ninety minutes. Overriding your BRAC too consistently leads to burnout because by going against your body's natural rhythm and staying in activation mode all the time, you are stimulating only the sympathetic branch of your nervous system. This, as explained earlier, creates stress on your overall nervous system and releases an abundance of cortisol, known as the stress hormone.

Mothers, especially with babies and young toddlers, override their BRAC all the time. They ignore their body's natural urge to rest because there are few opportunities in their day to rest. Working women do this too. Rachel, a woman in her early sixties and mother of teenage twins, worked privately with me for months. During our first visit, she confessed that while she loved her work and her children, it felt like the successful company she had built for three decades was killing her. She had fibromyalgia, a chronic disorder of pain and other symptoms, and now her doctors suspected she may have rheumatoid arthritis, an autoimmune disease of chronic inflammation. She told me she had not gotten a good night's sleep since her twins were born and had been on sleep medication for fifteen years, even though she knew it was bad for her health and probably not even working. It's impossible to know exactly why someone gets any disease, but it is clear that if we spend years overriding our body's natural need for rest, health issues can arise. In fact, Dr. Rubin Naiman calls depression "broken BRAC," or essentially staying in a state of activation without rest.[9]

The bottom line: it is not healthy to live in high-alert mode. Living well means living in harmony with our BRAC. We need to balance our high-alert periods with low-alert rest periods—opportunities for the parasympathetic branch of our nervous systems to kick in and for our cortisol levels to come back to healthy levels. The good news is that through the use of a yoga nidra nap, the Daring to Rest program will teach you how to take back your BRAC.

Rest Helps Us Cool Down

Science is showing that the planet is heating up, and perhaps not coincidentally, so are we. The explosion in the number of people experiencing autoimmune diseases, allergies, and other inflammation-related conditions suggests that people's systems are overheated. Eighty percent of people with autoimmune diseases today are women, and scientists cannot find clear reasons for this.[10] But in my experience, when I follow the trail of stressed-out women not getting good sleep, there are some compelling clues why this number is so high.

When we are truly resting, our core body temperature drops, and our brain goes into delta brain waves, which helps our organs regenerate. If you don't get good sleep or other types of rest, you don't cool down. And even if you do get good sleep, it might not be enough to counteract the effects of inflammation and overheating. The typical person consumes too much energy in daily life, and as a result, we have elevated heart rates, elevated cortisol levels, decreased melatonin levels, an overactive sympathetic nervous system, and an overactive hypothalamic-pituitary-adrenal (HTPA) axis, a major part of the neuroendocrine system that controls our reaction to stress, regulates digestion, the immune system, mood and emotions, and sexuality, not to mention the part of the brain that channels energy into consciousness. Truly restful practices, such as yoga nidra meditation, give our bodies the opportunity to cool down, as well as calm down.

Rest Connects Us with Our Deep Knowing

When life gets crazy busy, it's easy to lose a part of our creative, passionate, and instinctive self. Lack of rest is causing us to forget our instinctive, wilder nature. Jungian psychoanalyst Clarissa Pinkola Estés calls this a "female psychic slumber."[11] Men betray their instinctive nature too, but according to Estés, women will die if they lose touch with this deep, wild knowing. Women must connect to their inner world to redevelop this deep knowing, and rest can take us there because slowing down opens the door to this world. It's here you find your internal power switch, the "wild" you who doesn't run around like a robot or the good girl you were trained to be, following the masses when your gut tells you not to—and as a result, you wake from your slumber. Turning that switch back on is the goal of the Daring to Rest program.

2

WELCOME TO YOGA NIDRA

The first time I experienced yoga nidra, I fell in love, and here's why: I could lie down. It was as if *finally* I had been given permission to rest. I called it my adult nap. I made yoga nidra the centerpiece of my Daring to Rest program because it's the best tool I know to help people slow down, recover from burnout, and relieve stress. I can't wait for you to experience this "meditation with a cherry on top."

Why do I call yoga nidra that? Because meditation is typically practiced sitting upright, and during most types of meditation, you remain in waking state consciousness, sometimes focusing on a mantra or the breath. Yoga nidra, on the other hand, is typically practiced lying down, underneath a blanket, and it guides you from waking state to a dreaming state to a deep-sleep state and then beyond to a fourth state of consciousness where all thoughts stop. Without any effort, your mind goes into the deepest state of relaxation imaginable. Yoga nidra doesn't pick a fight with meditation. Both are great. But if yoga nidra gives you all the benefits of deep meditation *plus* the benefits of deep sleep, *and* you get to lie down while doing it, then to me it is clearly the hot-fudge sundae of meditation.

What Is Yoga Nidra?

Yoga nidra is a sleep-based, conscious relaxation and meditation technique. It is also known as *yogic sleep*. *Yoga* means "union" or "oneness" in Sanskrit, and *nidra* means "sleep," or more specifically, the consciousness that pervades all states, from waking to sleeping. In yoga nidra, you are guided into a sleep state but invited to remain conscious in a semi-awakened state while deeply relaxed. It's similar to a nap because you're asleep, but different because a typical nap shuts down everything, including awareness, while yoga nidra meditation guides you to shut down everything and *add* awareness. As a result, you become aware of different parts of the body, and relaxation is more effective. You also become open to erasing emotional and mental patterns that are holding you back.

Don't let the term *yoga* confuse you. There are no downward-facing dogs, warriors, or other physical poses in yoga nidra meditation. Instead, yoga nidra looks like an extension of *savasana*, or corpse pose, a pose you do at the end of most yoga classes where you lie down on the floor for rest and integration.

While the roots of yoga nidra are in ancient tantra yoga, a branch of Indian spiritual study, it was developed in the West for a mainstream audience in the 1960s by Swami Satyananda Saraswati of the Bihar School of Yoga. Decades earlier, as a student studying under a guru, Swami Satyananda says he fell asleep while a group of students chanted mantras nearby. Even though he was deeply asleep during the chanting, when he awoke, he could recall all of the mantras. His guru explained that this was because he had heard the mantras with his subtle body.

Swami Satyananda became curious and began to research what ancient tantric texts said about this awakening of the energy of this subtle body, a tantric process called *nysaa* (which in Sanskrit means "to take the mind to a point"). During nysaa, you bring your attention from one point in the body to another while you repeat a mantra to awaken subtle energy in the physical body. Seeking to develop the practice of nysaa for Westerners, Swami Satyananda got rid of the mantras (knowing most people in the West would be confused by them) but kept the principle of rotating consciousness throughout the body.

Today, the term *yoga nidra* typically refers to this conscious relaxation and meditation technique developed by Swami Satyananda, and its most defining feature is bringing attention to different layers of consciousness, from the most gross, like the physical body, to more and more subtle, nonphysical layers. Others have expanded and/or taken different approaches to yoga nidra over the years, such as Yogi Amrit Desai, who developed the Amrit Method of Yoga Nidra, and Richard Miller, who developed iRest meditation. But most yoga nidra approaches in the Western world have their roots in Swami Satyananda's method.

How Yoga Nidra Works

Okay, here's when I start shaking my yoga nidra pompoms. Yoga nidra is very simple: you simply lie on your back (or sit, if you prefer) and listen to the voice (either recorded or live) of the person leading the meditation. The voice prompts guide you from your crazy-busy outer life into your inner senses and into a relaxed, subconscious state of mind.

Typically, you are first invited to set an intention, known in Sanskrit as a *sankulpa*—a positive resolve, like a sacred vow you choose to focus on. I've devoted all of chapter four to setting your intention because it's such a powerful part of the yoga nidra process and the Daring to Rest program. After you say your intention, you are guided to rotate attention to different points throughout your physical body. Then you are guided to move through more subtle layers of yourself, using breathing techniques to relax and mindfulness techniques—including visualization, affirmations, and guided imagery—to dissolve limiting beliefs, lift heaviness from your body, and feel lighter and more peaceful.

What do I mean by moving through more subtle layers of yourself? We tend to think of ourselves as just our physical bodies, because this is what we see when we look in the mirror, but the yoga teachings on which yoga nidra is based tell us that we are actually made up of five bodies of awareness, known as *koshas* in Sanskrit:

The physical body

The energy body

The mental body

The wisdom body

The bliss body

The five-bodies model comes from the Upanishads, a collection of writings from ancient India that form the core of Indian philosophy and have been used as a yoga model for healing for thousands of years. The five bodies, or sheaths, are layered around the central true self, also known as the soul. The physical body is composed of physical matter, while the other four are composed of progressively more subtle layers of energy. If one or more of these bodies is not in balance, then illness or discord can arise.

In every yoga nidra meditation, you are guided to move your attention through all of these five bodies. You will learn more about each of them as you progress through the Daring to Rest program in chapters four through twelve. I like to think of the journey through the five bodies as a journey back to wholeness. Rotating attention to these bodies cleans your system of tension and stress. Imagine an onion and its layers; our five bodies are five layers of awareness that reside in us. The more you focus attention on them, the clearer they get, and the better you feel. They also point you to your true nature, which is essentially your most authentic self.

Pointing you to your most authentic self is the ultimate purpose of yoga nidra because that is where your internal power switch lies. In today's modern world, we're disconnected from our authentic self because we're fixated only on our physical body—through exercise, nutrition, weight loss, and health care, for example. The problem is, the physical body isn't where our internal power switch sits. Instead, accessing this power switch requires accessing all of your five bodies, and this allows your soul to fulfill its purpose.

The four subtle bodies (the energy, mental, wisdom, and bliss bodies) are what inspired Swami Satyananda to develop yoga nidra for modern times. He found that the more our awareness was directed to specific parts of the physical body, the more it relaxed, and relaxing the physical body opened a doorway to the other four bodies. Bringing attention to these more subtle bodies, in turn, increased the potential for deeper healing and rejuvenation in all parts of the physical body and the mind. Ultimately, yoga nidra meditation is a practice that takes you to a place of no stress because in the bliss body, you go into a timeless state, no longer chained to your to-do lists and obligations. Imagine just a few minutes each day when your mind powers down and does nothing—no thoughts, just open space, pure freedom. Rotating attention through five bodies is the road map to this space.

The yoga nidra meditations used in the Daring to Rest program guide your attention through each of the five bodies, helping you keep each one open and clear. In doing so, you begin to find your way back to that spark inside of you. You create the potential to flip your internal power switch back on, and this recharges your body, mind, spirit, and deep knowing.

Your Brain on Yoga Nidra

Each time you practice yoga nidra meditation, you're stilling the waves of the mind through conscious entry into the sleep state. How?

You start with sensing the body and breathing in specific ways in order to trigger the relaxation response. The relaxation response balances the sympathetic and parasympathetic nervous systems and balances the left and right brains. In the process, your brain shifts from beta, an awakened state with lots of brain activity, to alpha, a more relaxed state. In alpha, the mood-regulating hormone serotonin gets released, and this calms you down. People who spend little time in an alpha brain-wave state have more anxiety than those who spend more time in alpha. Think of a car: if you want to stop and turn off the engine, you first need to downshift. Shifting your brain into an alpha state starts its process of "powering down," or coming into a rest state with slower, restorative brain-wave activity.

From alpha, you go into a deep alpha and high theta brain-wave state—the dream state, REM sleep. In theta, your thoughts slow down to 4 to 8 thoughts per second. This is where superlearning happens. Kids and artists experience a lot more theta activity in their brains.

Emotional integration and release also happen here, and structures in the brain change. It's here that some people have random thoughts or see images. A person in theta may see colors or visions or hear the voice of a person talking, yet at the same time not hear this voice. It's where you begin to enter the gap of nothingness.

After theta, you are guided to delta, where your thoughts are only 1 to 3.9 thoughts per second. This is the most restorative state, in which your organs regenerate and the stress hormone cortisol is removed from your system.

When you're put under anesthesia, you're put into a delta brainwave state. Also, people in comas are in a delta brain-wave state, which gives their bodies a chance to restore their systems. In our culture, very few people go into the deep states of sleep like theta and delta on a regular basis, and as a consequence, our bodies are not powering down and getting the chance to restore themselves. Depressed people go to beta and alpha states, but rarely go to theta and delta.

From delta, the guided yoga nidra experience takes you down into an even deeper brain-wave state—one that can't be reached through conventional sleep. In this fourth state of consciousness, below delta, your brain is thoughtless. This state is sort of like a complete loss of consciousness, but you are awake. This state is one of such a deep surrender, where your consciousness is so far away from the physical body that living here every day would be difficult. Not everyone who practices yoga nidra touches this state, but the more you practice, the more you'll receive glimpses of it.

After you touch into the fourth state of consciousness, you are guided back to a waking state. Again, you couldn't live in this fourth state, but as a result of touching into it, you bring a little of its deep peace back with you to your waking, everyday brain state. You also are able to rewire your thoughts and emotions because your subconscious mind in this fourth state is fertile, more open to intentions and affirmations than it is when you are in your waking state. As a consequence, in your everyday life, you begin to rest more and more in the space between emotions and thoughts, and resting in this space gives rise to a sense of freedom, where you are not triggered so much by the stuff in your life.

Throughout the yoga nidra meditation I will teach you, you are often asked to bring your attention to the space between your eyebrows—a spot known as the third eye. Behind this spot lies the pineal gland, and this gland is stimulated when you bring your attention there. Studies confirm that the pineal-gland hormone, melatonin, is a powerful agent for reducing stress, inducing more restful sleep, and boosting the immune system, which helps prevent illness, promote healing, and slow premature aging.

Benefits of Yoga Nidra

While yoga nidra is not a substitute for sleep, the number-one reason most women I know say yes to yoga nidra is that it's widely touted that forty-five minutes of yogic sleep feels like three hours of regular sleep. There's some debate over the science that backs this up, but it is likely this effect is due to the series of brain-wave changes experienced during yoga nidra.[1] In my work, I hear women tell me all the time that they wake up deeply refreshed after practicing yoga nidra and that yoga nidra helps them fall asleep and get back to sleep at night. Who can say no to sleep?

As you can imagine, feeling well rested is life changing, but yoga nidra also improves your overall health. A 2011 study showed that practicing yoga nidra improved anxiety, depression, and overall well-being for women having menstrual irregularities and psychological problems.[2] I've worked with many women who have had tremendous success using yoga nidra to help them manage anxiety and pain, which has also been noted by Kamakhya Kumar in *A Handbook of Yoga Nidra*.[3] And even more science points to how yoga nidra can help lower blood pressure and cholesterol, and improve blood glucose fluctuations and symptoms associated with diabetes.[4]

The explosion of studies supporting the benefits of meditation also apply to yoga nidra because yoga nidra is a form of meditation. Both meditation and yoga nidra help activate the relaxation response and improve the functioning of your nervous system and endocrine system, which affects your hormones. Both meditation and yoga nidra help cells regenerate and repair, and both help decrease anxiety and improve your mood.

Women tell me all the time how practicing yoga nidra meditation has positively impacted their family life. One mother who was checked out of her life due to exhaustion now practices yoga nidra and says that she is using more loving speech to herself, her children, and her spouse and is parenting from a more peaceful place. Another woman who felt imprisoned by her anxiety tells me she is now able to lead a full life with her family from a calm place. It's clear to me that women get their family and freedom back when they practice yoga nidra regularly.

One yoga teacher told me that yoga nidra planted a seed in her to rest and practice kindness toward herself. She had always taught her students about the value of rest and kindness, but ironically, she found it challenging to give herself either. She told me that by practicing one yoga nidra meditation at a time, she noticed how everything in her body felt as if it flowed better and how her mind became clearer. Another woman—a mother, entrepreneur, and writer with an autoimmune disorder and crippling fatigue—told me that once everyone in her family is out of the house in the morning, she practices yoga nidra "around the time a newborn would take her first nap." This regular practice of yoga nidra began shifting something inside her, renewing her energy and ability to focus, and boosting her drive to get to work on her projects that matter. I hear this same theme from women all the time, even in quite challenging circumstances: how yoga nidra feels like a magical force helping them feel deeply rested, focused, and then able to rise to a better place.

What You Need to Practice Yoga Nidra

The only essentials you'll need to practice yoga nidra are (1) a yoga nidra meditation audio, (2) a means of listening to that audio, and (3) a place to rest, ideally lying down. There are no expensive props, and you can practice yoga nidra meditation in virtually any quiet space. For years, I regularly did yoga nidra parked in my minivan during my younger son's soccer practice, reclining the front seat, putting in earbuds, and plugging into a yoga nidra meditation audio on my smartphone.

There are optional props that you might want to use to make your yoga nidra more relaxing. I'm a huge fan of using an eye pillow because it can help relax tension in your head and provide complete darkness. If you're doing yoga nidra on an airplane or in a loud home (such as in an apartment in a city or when there are lots of kids at home), you might choose to use earbuds plugged into an MP3 player or smartphone. It's also nice to have a blanket (or at least a sweater) because warmth helps you relax, and when you lie down, you tend to lose heat. Although some people won't use a pillow under their heads, I find it's okay to use one if you feel you need neck support. Also, you may want to put pillows or a bolster under your knees to support your lower back.

Do you *have* to have a place to lie down when practicing yoga nidra? No. You can practice yoga nidra just as effectively when sitting upright in a chair. I practice yoga nidra leaning slightly back in airplane or bus seats all the time. If you're in an office and can close your door, you can practice while sitting in your chair.

Many people ask me where they should lie down to practice yoga nidra, and I tell them anywhere that's comfortable. If you take a yoga nidra class at a yoga studio, as I first did, you'll probably be lying on a yoga mat with a blanket over your body. You can certainly do the same thing at home or in other settings, but you don't have to lie on a yoga mat. In fact, I rarely do. At home, most people practice their yoga nidra while lying on a carpeted floor, on a couch, or on a bed.

Sometimes I practice yoga nidra in my bed before going to sleep at night or in the morning when I wake up. Practicing while in bed works for many, but not all people. If you have sleep issues and are not planning to go directly to sleep after your yoga nidra practice, listening to yoga nidra meditations while lying in your regular bed may not be the best option. Instead, try lying on a different bed or on your couch and doing yoga nidra outside of your regular sleep times. Let your intuition and experiences guide you.

Yoga nidra doesn't take a lot of time. Listening to a yoga nidra meditation typically takes from twenty to forty minutes. The three yoga nidra meditations I've designed for the Daring to Rest program take about fifteen minutes, thirty minutes, and forty minutes, respectively. (Chapter three will tell you where and how to access these recorded Daring to Rest yoga nidra meditations or record them yourself.) So take "I'm too busy" out of your vocabulary. Most people can find pockets of time, whether it's during a lunch break at work or before going to bed.

One single mom initially told me that there was no time in her day to practice yoga nidra, and she was too tired at night and got up too early in the morning to practice. My response to this problem is to be creative and to trust that kids above the age of eight (and even younger, sometimes) can be trained to respect your yoga nidra time. We decided that when she returned home from work, she would spend fifteen minutes catching up with the kids, and then before cooking dinner, she would take her twenty-minute yoga nidra nap. She told her kids that this was the new routine, and the kids made a "Mommy's napping" sign for her door. If the sign was on the door, they were not to enter. If children are under eight, I normally tell moms to allow them to enter quietly to lie down beside you if they need to and see how it goes. Some kids can do it, others can't. In her situation, within a week her kids were trained. She got her yoga nidra nap, and then she could continue her evening with the kids, feeling recharged.

What usually happens after women create a new yoga nidra routine is that yoga nidra time very quickly becomes nonnegotiable. It's something they know they need. And everyone in the household also begins demanding that these women take their yoga nidra nap because the family sees the incredible results.

Frequently Asked Questions

You may have more questions about yoga nidra before or as you begin doing yoga nidra. Here are the questions I most frequently hear from women and the answers I give.

What If I fall asleep while doing yoga nidra? Falling asleep is actually quite common the first few times people practice yoga nidra. If you do fall asleep, it's okay; your subconscious mind will still receive the instructions, and you will benefit because yoga nidra speaks to the part of you that never sleeps. But ideally you don't want to sleep. So try practicing yoga nidra while seated in a chair—maybe do it this way for a week—and then, when you stop falling asleep, return to doing yoga nidra lying down. Sitting in a chair sends a signal to most bodies to stay awake.

Many times people think they have fallen asleep during yoga nidra, but they haven't. You know you've fallen asleep if at the end of the meditation you do not wake up. If, however, you think you fell asleep, but you wake up at the end when prompted to wake, then you were most likely not asleep. Instead, you were deeply relaxed, often in a very deep state of meditation.

Is yoga nidra safe if I've experienced trauma? Multiple preliminary studies of iRest yoga nidra, a type of yoga nidra developed by Richard Miller, show that it significantly reduces symptoms and is a promising integrative therapy for women with sexual trauma.[5] While the yoga nidra I teach isn't strictly the iRest protocol, yoga nidra meditation is normally a safe practice for people with trauma, and many people, including me, have shifted out of trauma using yoga nidra. But if you have experienced or are experiencing severe trauma, it's best to consult your medical provider before beginning to practice yoga nidra. Also, yoga nidra does not replace any needed therapy or medication.

If you have experienced trauma, it is important to imagine a safe space in your mind before you practice yoga nidra. This can be a quiet place in nature or at the home of someone who loves you deeply. It can also be an imagined place that you have not experienced, like beside a waterfall or in a calming blue room. Really feel as if you are in this space; experience the smells, the air, all the details of the environment. Then each time you practice yoga nidra, you can go to this safe space if you start to feel unsafe in any way. In iRest yoga nidra, Richard Miller calls this safe place "your inner resource."[6]

Throughout the Daring to Rest program, I encourage you to use a touchstone during yoga nidra as your safety tool. You can read more about this in chapter three.

Is yoga nidra safe if I have a serious medical condition? If you have a serious medical condition, always check in with your medical care provider and yourself before starting a yoga nidra meditation practice. While yoga nidra is safe for most people, only you and your medical support people know your unique situation.

Is yoga nidra safe if I have a sleep disorder? You may greatly benefit from practicing yoga nidra meditation if you have sleep issues, such as trouble getting to sleep or getting back to sleep after waking during the night. During the Daring to Rest program, you will be asked to practice yoga nidra each day but not in the middle of the night. If you want to use yoga nidra to help you get back to sleep after waking up at night, you can use the same yoga nidra meditation an additional time. You don't want to train your body to expect yoga nidra in the middle of the night.

Also, if you have sleep issues and practice yoga nidra during the day, ideally practice in a place that's not your bed. That way, you'll keep your bed a place for sleeping only.

What if my mind has lots of thoughts during yoga nidra? It's common for lots of thoughts to flood your mind as soon as you lie down—everything from your to-do list to random thoughts. If this happens, try to focus on the guided instructions of the yoga nidra meditation. This can often help distract your mind from thoughts, so you can let them go.

What if I feel lots of sensations like emotions or pain during yoga nidra? Yoga nidra is a beautiful process that invites you to welcome all sensations in your body. Occasionally, you may feel sensations so deeply that it is uncomfortable. If you continue to stay with these feelings, nonjudgmentally, often you will feel a shift to a more comfortable place. If you don't, and instead you feel these sensations shifting you to an even less comfortable place, first try squeezing your touchstone (explained in chapter three). You can also imagine a safe space in your mind, a place where you feel totally at ease, and go there. How to shift to a safe space is described in more detail under the earlier question, "Is yoga nidra safe if I've experienced trauma?"

What if I need to scratch an itch or move during yoga nidra? Can I do so? Yes, absolutely. But if you need to move, do it mindfully—slowly and with full awareness. The point is to be comfortable while doing yoga nidra, and moving quickly or suddenly can startle you out of a deeply relaxed state.

How do I practice yoga nidra if I have small children? I started practicing yoga nidra when my kids were two and four—not ages that easily allow Mom to get quiet time. If you have a baby, you may want to practice while the baby is napping in another room; when you're sitting in a chair and breastfeeding (a great time for you and the baby!); at bedtime, just after the baby has gone to bed; or early morning, before the baby wakes.

With toddlers and young children, you can take your yoga nidra nap at the same time as your kids' regular nap. Also, as I mentioned earlier, try putting a sign on the door to your bedroom or practice area, and tell older children that when the sign is up, Mommy's taking her (yoga nidra) nap. If they see that sign, they are not to disturb you.

Some young children are happy to lie down with you and listen to yoga nidra. This wasn't possible with my older son, but my younger son loved to come in to lie down when I was doing yoga nidra. I like to ring a singing bowl before I begin my yoga nidra meditation and again at the end; when my son was with me, I'd let him ring my singing bowl. He loved that role. As he got older, he understood that if he could not wait until the end of the yoga nidra to move, he was to go into the other room and play until I was done; he could not play in the yoga nidra nap room. Most kids are very trainable to honor your yoga nidra time, but you must be clear and consistent with the boundaries, so everyone's happy.

Is yoga nidra hypnosis? No, yoga nidra is not hypnosis. While there are some similarities, the purpose of hypnosis is to create shifts in the mind/body. In yoga nidra, the purpose is for you to rediscover the truth of who you are, your true nature. Shifts in mind/body do occur, but that's not the purpose of yoga nidra. All changes within you happen spontaneously as a result of releasing stress and tension, as well as the intention you set. Also, hypnosis involves more of a switching off of the left side of the brain and letting the right side take over. Yoga nidra has clear rotations through the left and right sides of the brain, which gives rise to a state of oneness. From oneness, you feel well rested, you notice rhythm and resonance in your life, and you make changes in alignment with your heart's desire.

3

THE DARING TO REST
PROGRAM

Imagine spending forty days to reboot your system on physical, mental, emotional, spiritual, and energetic levels and, in doing so, laying the groundwork for a well-rested life moving forward. This is the goal of the Daring to Rest program: to create an oasis for you to break the cycle of fatigue and, from a well-rested place, to gain the courage to lead a life full of purpose.

Three Phases: Rest, Release, Rise

The program is divided into three phases, reflecting the three key Daring to Rest principles. These principles, the heart of the Daring to Rest philosophy, will guide you throughout the program. I also think of them as the three layers of exhaustion women hold. Through yoga nidra meditation, and other optional practices, the Daring to Rest program helps you shine awareness and effectively clean up each layer of exhaustion.

Rest: Physical exhaustion. The first layer of exhaustion we explore is in the body and our energetic field, because exhaustion often feels physical. If you don't get enough rest, your body will be tired. The emphasis during this phase is to deeply relax and start sleeping better. Rest is always the first step to wellness. It is essential in good health and sleep, and for women, it's an opportunity to reconnect to our desires, regulate our cycles, and shed physical exhaustion.

Release: Emotional exhaustion. The second layer of exhaustion is emotional. Have you been holding on to feelings and thoughts that no longer serve you? You're not alone. This is common, which is why during this phase, simply by practicing yoga nidra meditation, you will begin to release self-defeating emotions and thoughts such as the feeling of not being enough or anger that's turned into rage. You'll experience how yoga nidra meditation helps you release these exhausting emotions and thoughts, and you'll unleash a wild part of your nature that's been yearning for your attention. (Yes, major pompom shakes!)

Rise: Life-purpose exhaustion. Not following your life purpose? Don't even know what it is? Yep, that's exhausting. In this final phase, I show you how to take your yoga nidra meditation into the real world and be a well-rested leader. Most women don't lead to become rich; we lead to fulfill our purpose on the planet. Our leadership may include financial abundance, but typically money is not what ultimately fuels us. If you're not feeling full of purpose, this final phase will help clear that exhaustion. It will get you on track to a fully rebooted and well-rested life after you've finished the program.

Key Features of the Daring to Rest Program

Whether you have practiced yoga nidra before or not, there are some defining features of the Daring to Rest program that make this a unique yoga nidra experience. Here are a few important details you should know before getting started.

Yoga Nidra Meditations

I've created three custom yoga nidra meditations for the Daring to Rest program, one for each phase:

Phase One: Rest Meditation

Phase Two: Release Meditation

Phase Three: Rise Meditation

You can download my recordings of all three, free, from the *Daring to Rest* page on the Sounds True website: SoundsTrue.com/daringtorest/yoganidrameditations. Simply load them onto your smartphone or MP3 player, turn the meditation on, lie down, and rest.

You can also record the yoga nidra meditations on your own, using the scripts and instructions provided in appendix 1, at the back of the book.

Soul Whispers

In the Daring to Rest yoga nidra meditations, I prompt you to listen for a soul whisper every time you practice yoga nidra. Why? Because one of the biggest reasons we stay worn out is a chronic disconnection from our souls. The soul is the seat of your true power; it's where your internal power switch resides and reminds you that you are endowed with all the resources to succeed. This program is about turning on that power switch, which is why I want you to track your soul whispers for the forty days. Soul whispers give us clues to how we're really feeling under the "busy" coats we wear every day.

Finding your soul whisper takes only a minute or two at the end of yoga nidra meditation. You'll breathe in through your heart, imagine your breath guiding you to an area of your body, and then see if there is a word, image, or phrase that appears. After you finish your meditation, write down what you received. If you get nothing, that's okay; write down the word *nothing*. The important point is to let yourself be led to your soul whisper through feeling, not thinking.

I ask you to listen for your soul whisper at the end of yoga nidra meditation because yoga nidra takes you deep into your inner world, where you can clearly hear the voice of your soul, and this gives you a better understanding of what you are feeling and your true heart-based desires. For many of us, it's not easy to hear a soul whisper in our everyday lives. With practice, you'll be able to tap into your soul whisper anywhere, but the ideal place to start listening to this whisper is at the end of yoga nidra meditation because yoga nidra is a pointer back to your soul.

Power Centers

As explained in chapter two, yoga nidra meditation guides you through what are known as the five bodies: the physical body and four bodies of subtle energy that encase your soul in layers. In each of the three Daring to Rest yoga nidra meditations, I also guide you to specific *power centers*. In Sanskrit, these energetic power centers are known as *chakras*. The seven major power centers follow a path from your root (base of your spine) to the crown of your head. They are centers of transformation that turn psychophysical energy into spiritual energy, enabling you to feel whole. Focusing on these power centers gives you a way to focus on different areas of your body while you practice yoga nidra meditation. When attempting to release blocked energy from your five bodies, it's helpful to work with the related power centers, both during yoga nidra and in your everyday life, as they help bring peace and balance.

A Touchstone

When you start practicing yoga nidra, you begin to clear emotions and thoughts that you've spent a lifetime identifying with but that no longer support your well-being. As a result, you might experience "detox" symptoms similar to the physical symptoms we experience when doing an internal cleanse. Emotional and mental detox symptoms can range from crying to simply being more aware of feeling than usual because the worn-out woman often gets quite good at numbing herself to feeling.

To help you navigate such symptoms over the next forty days, I want you to find a small object, a touchstone. You can keep it beside you when you practice yoga nidra meditation, or hold it in your left hand (your feminine side). Many women use objects from nature, like a small shell they found on vacation on the beach or a stone from their favorite hiking trail. Others use touchstones that have more literal meaning, like a special ring from a deceased grandmother or a crystal. You can place your touchstone on different body parts while you practice yoga nidra meditation; I'll tell you more about this in each chapter.

You can also keep your touchstone in your pocket or purse, put it on an altar in the room where you practice yoga nidra, or put it in another special place to touch whenever you feel the worn-out woman returning. This touchstone will reconnect you to your well-rested woman and a feeling of safety in the body.

The majority of people who practice yoga nidra don't feel intense emotions at all. In fact, they feel exactly the opposite: they feel calmer than ever. If that's the case for you, it's still important to use your touchstone because it reminds you, when your worn-out woman wants to come back in, that everything is going to be okay. I remember when a woman in the Daring to Rest program told me that she was on her own on an airplane with her four kids, and her youngest was screaming from the time they boarded the plane. It was horrible, but she told me that the moment she took out her touchstone, her energy shifted, and she remembered, "Oh yes, I am okay." Your touchstone helps you hear your well-rested woman, connecting you to that calm yoga nidra voice that knows everything is going to be okay.

How Your Forty Days Will Go

Your primary instruction throughout the forty-day Daring to Rest program is to practice yoga nidra meditation every day and listen for your soul whisper. Ideally, I would like you to listen to the Daring to Rest meditations I've created for this program because they are designed specifically to complement the content of the chapters. If you have a different yoga nidra meditation you prefer listening to, go ahead, but please be sure to spend a minute or two listening for your soul whisper on your own at the end of the meditation and then track it in a journal.

As you move through this book, here's how the forty days will break down:

Phase	Days	Chapters	Yoga Nidra Meditation
Rest	1–5	Chapter Four: Intention	Phase One: Rest Meditation (15 min.)
	6–10	Chapter Five: Body	Phase One: Rest Meditation (15 min.)
	11–15	Chapter Six: Energy	Phase One: Rest Meditation (15 min.)
Release	16–20	Chapter Seven: Mind	Phase Two: Release Meditation (30 min.)
	21–25	Chapter Eight: Wisdom	Phase Two: Release Meditation (30 min.)
	26–30	Chapter Nine: Bliss	Phase Two: Release Meditation (30 min.)
Rise	31–35	Chapter Ten: Lead	Phase Three: Rise Meditation (40 min.)
	36–40	Chapter Eleven: Life	Phase Three: Rise Meditation (40 min.)

Chapters four through eleven guide you through the Daring to Rest program. Each chapter focuses on different themes, the five bodies, and each chapter offers additional, optional practices you can use to supplement the yoga nidra meditations and customize your Daring to Rest experience.

At the end of each chapter, optional prompts invite you to dive deeper into the themes of the chapter. You can respond to these prompts with freewriting (described below under "Keep a Journal"), discussing them in a group, or through movement. Choose a prompt that speaks to you. To begin your response, put your hand over your heart; take a slow, deep breath; repeat the prompt; and then begin writing, talking, moving, or responding in your own way.

I encourage you to move through your forty-day journey chapter by chapter and not jump ahead or follow instructions out of order. You can read through the entire book first if this helps motivate you, but then do the program in order without skipping any instructions. So, you'll read one chapter, practice yoga nidra meditation for five days, and then move on. In each phase, you will increase the amount of time you listen to yoga nidra meditation.

Tips for Successfully Completing the Program

While practicing yoga nidra meditation is simple and easy to do, the reality is, we lead busy lives. The women who have the most success with the Daring to Rest program intentionally create space in their lives to make it happen. Here are some tips to help you get the most out of the program.

Schedule it. Decide when you will practice yoga nidra meditation and put it on your calendar for the next forty days. The best time to practice is when it's the most convenient for you, but many women like to practice in either the morning, upon waking, or just before bed. Write it down. I even tell women to write "physical therapy" in their calendars if this will help them take rest more seriously. If you can, build in fifteen minutes before and after your yoga nidra practice for any complementary practices like journaling or for transition time.

Set up a designated space to rest. While you can practice yoga nidra virtually anywhere, and you don't need any fancy props, when you are at home, it is ideal to have a specific place to rest. This is your rest cave. It's a quiet place where you can drop the worn-out woman. It is also a fertile place where you can give birth to things—new ideas, new plans, and new yearnings. Be creative with your rest cave. Some women string lights to turn on after yoga nidra to journal. Others use a special blanket.

Create a rest altar. An altar gives you a place in your home where you can honor rest, come back to your center, and welcome your well-rested woman. This altar is where you can put meaningful items like your touchstone, any essential oils you may choose to use with your yoga nidra practice, a journal for recording your soul whispers, or any other object that sings to your heart. Your rest cave, or wherever you typically will practice yoga nidra meditation, is a great place for an altar. You can also use a beautiful tray as your altar and move it around your home.

Keep a journal. From tracking your soul whispers to responding to the optional prompts in each chapter, a journal keeps your notes from your Daring to Rest journey in one place. This is where you can do any optional freewriting. To freewrite, first choose to write for either three minutes or three pages, and then keep your hand writing the whole time. If you cannot think of anything to write, then write "nothing," or write your current soul whisper again and again until you do have something to write. This is intuitive writing—the key is to get out of your head, let yourself be "wild," and write anything, even if it surprises you.

Get your family on board. One of the biggest obstacles to success is a family that is unwilling to give you the space to rest. Before you start the program, tell them you're making this forty-day commitment and ask for their support to protect your time to rest. If you have young kids and can't figure out how to rest with them home, find them care outside the home or ask another mom to do a childcare swap. (For more tips for practicing yoga nidra when you have young children, see the "Frequently Asked Questions" section in chapter two.)

Chuck perfect. Women always ask me, "What if I miss a day during the forty-day program?" Do I have to go back to the beginning? No. You chuck perfect and keep going. Don't skip the activities for the day you missed; just continue with the program right where you left off on the day you begin again. Ideally, you'll need to miss or skip only a day or two, for special events or emergencies. So you will practice forty days of yoga nidra meditation, but it may take you forty-five days.

"Chuck perfect" is the motto this program lives by. Perfectionism has held women back and burnt us out for centuries. This program is not about doing it perfectly, but about making a deep commitment to be good to yourself. That doesn't mean you should finish the forty days in six months—that's not the kind of chucking perfect I mean. Chucking perfect is giving yourself permission to not rest for a day or two if you need to skip it, but then picking yourself back up soon after and getting back to a program that is designed to support your well-being.

Your Peaceful Oasis

How can this program create permanent shifts in your life? I will show you throughout this book, but very simply, yoga nidra helps you attune to your aliveness. It reminds you of what's important and gives you the courage and energy to stand in your purpose and remember that you are whole. You are enough. Yoga nidra is like hopping on a cruise ship to wholeness.

The women who immerse themselves in the Daring to Rest program understand this in every nerve and cell of their bodies and minds, and they take their wholeness back into the world in action-oriented ways as well-rested women. The model of the worn-out woman isn't an option anymore, or at least not for long, because after women complete this program, they know in their hearts that they don't want to live their lives as worn-out women. Worn out is clearly unsustainable. That's why the Daring to Rest program will affect all areas of your life, from work to home. As a mother from Montreal told me, yoga nidra is her "peaceful place," her "oasis" to go to. I encourage you to think of yoga nidra meditation this way too, as your peaceful oasis that you will get to visit regularly over the next forty days. You deserve this, Sister.

Phase One

REST

Permission to rest is granted.

Sleep specialist Rubin Naiman, PhD, points out, "Rest is a universal and critical ingredient in virtually all approaches to healing."[1] Yet today it's rare to meet someone who rests when they get sick, let alone when they're simply tired. Instead of lying down and doing nothing when we're exhausted, we try to do one more something—get more exercise, meet a friend for dinner, work late.

After just one time practicing my new yoga nidra nap, I saw this "do something" mind-set for what it truly is: bizarre. What crazy person doesn't rest when they're tired? I put my kids down for a nap every day to keep them from feeling exhausted. Why not me? Why was I grabbing for so many remedies, even healthy remedies like high-powered yoga workouts and green smoothies, to rescue me when rest was the most obvious remedy? Why don't we just rest when we're tired?

When you begin daring to rest with yoga nidra, the most immediate result you will feel is complete physical restoration of your body. The first time I practiced yoga nidra, it felt as if my body had caught up on all the sleep I'd been missing from the previous week. Lying there, under my blanket in the yoga studio, I began to deeply unwind, perhaps for the first time ever. In later sessions, I would be so relaxed at the end that sometimes I'd wake with a tear in my eye. Could I really feel this peaceful?

People laugh when I tell them I help women feel well rested. "Can you teach rest?" they ask, the assumption being that rest is something we all know how to do. But this is not true. Rest is something we have forgotten how to do and must relearn. Here in phase one, you have the opportunity to do just that—relearn how to rest.

My first daring-to-rest moment was the seed that blossomed into a regular yoga nidra practice, which has become a foundation in my life. I hear this echoed by women who have been in my yoga nidra programs, like Maria, who told me, "Yoga nidra meditation is now as foundational to me as drinking water, eating leafy greens, and exercising." That's the second thing this phase will teach you: how to start making rest a foundation in your life.

The more you rest, the better you will feel. And the better you feel, the easier it is to navigate times of transition or difficulty, like menstruation, fertility, pregnancy, motherhood, menopause, divorce, trauma, and grief.

What else can you expect to receive from regularly practicing yoga nidra meditation? Here is what women have told me:

> It deepens my understanding of quiet and gives perspective to my day.

> It takes my mind off the swirl, so I can go back to sleep.

> It keeps my container full and radiant because life doesn't slow down when you don't sleep.

> Now I'm so in touch with my body and the messages it sends out. . . . Taking the ritual of yoga nidra into my night routine completely shifted my sleep.

For the first five days of phase one, the focus is on setting an intention. This is important because living with intention is often the first thing to drop off our priority list when we get busy. As you'll learn in chapter four, an intention is the seed for everything that follows, including recovering from your physical exhaustion and breaking the cycle of fatigue. With yoga nidra, you'll get the benefit of coming into alignment with your heart's deepest intention—while at the same time, you get to lie down and take a restful nap. What could be easier than that?

4

INTENTION

Aligning with Your Heart's Desires

Days 1–5

During a yoga nidra meditation, you are prompted to state an *intention*—a positive resolve that gives purpose and meaning to your life. Sometimes you say your intention at the beginning of a yoga nidra meditation, but you always repeat it toward the end, when you're in the deepest state of consciousness, because that's when the subconscious mind is open. Planting an intention here is like planting a seed in fertile soil. Your mind is so still that there are virtually no thoughts to self-sabotage your intention. So the moment you repeat it, your mind absorbs it without question. The results are like magic; you begin to see unhelpful habits and patterns shift in your life and align with your stated intention. Because the intention is planted so deeply in your consciousness, whenever something in your daily life begins to shift out of alignment with it, you will feel a tug pulling you back to it.

For these first five days, you'll be resting deeply with yoga nidra meditation and discovering your intention for the Daring to Rest journey ahead. You'll be getting used to listening for soul whispers, a voice from your soul that's hard to hear in your everyday life, at the end of your yoga nidra practice.

Basic Instructions for Days 1 to 5

1. Practice the Phase One: Rest Meditation daily for five days. Be sure to hold your touchstone in your left hand or keep it nearby as you do the meditation.

2. Discover your intention by tracking your soul whispers, asking for one to three intention words, and creating a concise statement using these words.

3. Optional: Process concepts from this chapter with prompts to help you dive deeper into your intention, soul whispers, and rest.

Discovering Your Intention

Your intention is a statement that captures your heart's deepest desires for your life at this moment. It's like the trunk of a tree, growing out of the deep, strong roots of your heart. Think of your intention as a prayer: a short, powerful statement that comes from your heart and supports your total well-being.

An intention has the following qualities:

- It is one sentence and concise.

- It is stated in the present tense.

- It is always positive.

- It resonates deeply.

- It is not dependent on outcome.

Here are some examples of intentions from women in my programs:

I am loving and loved.

I trust life.

I am calm, joyful, and carefree.

I feel.

I am enough, I have enough, and I do enough.

I am patient and loving to myself and others.

As you rest throughout the next forty days, think of your intention as the seed you wish to plant for your life. It's not a goal. It's important to know that yoga nidra intentions are not dependent on outcome. That's where an intention differs from a goal. You're not willing something to happen; you're putting out a statement of what your heart desires, to bring you more in alignment with your most authentic self.

For example, "I am patient and loving to myself and others" is the intention used by a woman who had made an overseas move and had a baby. Now her baby was getting older, and she was finally taking a breath to ask herself, "What am I doing in my life?" Rather than focusing on a goal she wanted in her life, her intention didn't state a desired outcome; instead, it was a positive statement of how she wanted to *feel* toward herself (and others) during a big transition time. And it was stated in the present tense, as if she were already feeling it. The two important points are that she did not discover this intention from her head and that she claimed her intention as if it were already happening.

There are questions you can ask yourself to *think* your intention, like "Where am I stuck in life?" and "What do I need to feel unstuck?" but I would never tell you to make an intention only from your head. Why not? Because yoga nidra intentions don't come from your head; they come from your heart. They come from listening—listening deeply—to your soul. They address the "why."

A typical challenge women have when creating an intention statement is stating it in the present tense. Imagine stating, "I feel worthy," when that's what you feel the least at the moment. An intention often needs tweaking until you get it both positive and present. One woman told me her intention was "I can enjoy the life that I have created." I suggested she tweak the intention by taking out "can" and simply stating, "I enjoy the life that I have created." She explained that the reason she chose the word *can* was because "it feels like I'm giving myself permission." It's important to remember that an intention doesn't give you permission; instead, it is phrased as if you have already granted yourself permission. It's a statement phrased as if the choice has been made to live in alignment with your intention. I know this phrasing can feel uncomfortable if what your intention is saying is not yet true. Try to think of your intention as a seed you're planting. You're not planting permission for the seed to grow; you're planting exactly what you want to grow, so your intention is stated as if it's already happening. Then you need to water the seed. That's what yoga nidra meditation will do: your yoga nidra practice gives your intention permission to grow. This is similar to repeating an affirmation in the mirror—you repeat it as if it were true until you feel it.

You may already have an intention in mind after reading the beginning of this chapter or you may have had one when you bought this book. Even if that's the case, please follow the three steps outlined in the following sections to discover your intention during these first five days of your Daring to Rest program. Because your ideal intention is not necessarily the one you have in *mind*; it's the one lying awake in your heart and soul, the one speaking to you through your soul whispers, as described in chapter three.

Step One: Record Your Soul Whispers for Four Days

In this step, you'll listen to your soul whispers to help you identify your intention.

For the first four days of this program, you will practice the Phase One: Rest Meditation. When you are prompted to repeat an intention,

please say, "I am a well-rested woman," or any intention that spontaneously arises. At the end, you will be guided to listen for your soul whisper.

After finishing the meditation, write your soul whisper in a journal.
If you receive a soul whisper that doesn't make sense to you, don't
worry. Just write it down. There's no need to try to decode your soul
whispers. The most important thing is listening for them because, in
doing so, you're reestablishing the lines of communication between
your inner and outer worlds. You're also tapping into how in or out
of rhythm you feel. Recording them may allow you to see patterns or
messages later, as you continue your Daring to Rest program.

Sometimes soul whispers do not come as words, but as images,
sounds, or even something else, like a scent, a song, or an emotion.
Many women who are artists get soul whispers that are images. One
woman told me she once heard the sound of cows being milked in the
early morning, a familiar sound from her childhood. Be open to your
soul whisper coming through in both expected and unexpected ways.
The key is to keep your senses open and *feel* your soul whisper, which is
exactly what the Daring to Rest yoga nidra meditations guide you to do.

It is not uncommon to get nothing at least one of the days, or even
every day, because modern life doesn't prepare us to tap into our souls
easily. When we've lived as the worn-out woman for so long, many
times we've gone numb to feeling and hearing our inner world. That's
okay; these are just the first few days of this program. There is no pressure to achieve anything. Enjoy the rest!

If you received nothing when you asked for a soul whisper, then
write "nothing" in your journal for that day. I assure you that you'll
eventually get more than "nothing" for your soul whispers. And "nothing" is always something.

Step Two: Notice Words that
Resonate from Your Soul Whispers

On day five, write your four soul whispers on four pieces of paper. Even
if all of your papers say "nothing," write the word "nothing." If your soul
whisper was not a word or phrase, write down key words that describe

your soul whisper. If it was a song, write down the name of the song or lyrics that stood out. When you lie down to do your day 5 yoga nidra meditation, place all four soul whispers at the crown of your head.

At the end of the meditation, lay all four slips of paper in front of you face up, plus your day 5 soul whisper, and then close your eyes, put your hand over your heart, and breathe in and out once or twice through your heart. Now open your eyes, read each soul whisper, and notice one to three words from your soul whispers that resonate the most. Don't overthink this. If you can't make a decision, then turn the pieces of paper over so that you can't see them, close your eyes, shuffle, and with your left hand (your feminine, receiving hand) pick one to three pieces of paper. Trust that you always get what you need, even if it surprises you.

Worthy, possibility, peaceful, and *courageous* are just some of the soul whispers women I've worked with have received. Whatever you get, you will use these words to create your intention through the rest of phase one. In the Release and Rise phases, you'll have the option to change your intention, but only if it feels right.

It's important that your words be positive. If one of your words feels negative, then consider using the opposite of that word. For example, if you receive the word *war,* change it to *peace.* If your word was *nothing,* change it to *everything* or *something* if this feels positive. Also, if you do freewriting in your journal after you receive a soul whisper, as mentioned in the "Optional: Diving Deeper" section at the end of this chapter, look at your freewriting to see what words resonate for you. This can also inform your intention and help you find words that feel positive.

If none of the words from your soul whispers feels right, that's okay. Your intention may not be ready to present itself. If it feels right, you can use the placeholder word *rest* because rest is most likely why you picked up this book.

Step Three: Create Your Intention Statement

Right after you discover your one to three words, put an "I am," "I" or "I feel" in front of them and read the resulting sentence aloud. Then tap a few times on your heart with the index and middle fingers of your right hand and ask yourself, "Do I feel a yes when I read this statement?" If you do, this is your intention. For example, if your words were *safe* and *calm*, your intention would be "I am calm and safe" or "I feel calm and safe." Those phrases are great intention statements.

Depending on your words, you may need to tweak the wording a bit to achieve the best intention statement. For example, if you are using the word *rest*, you might want to consider saying, "I am well rested" or "I am a well-rested woman." One woman got *family* as her only word, and it didn't make sense to say, "I am family." So she reviewed the words she got from her soul whispers freewriting and saw the word *embrace*, which felt right in her heart. Her intention became "I embrace my family." You may need to use connector words like this.

Think of your intention statement as capturing a quality or state of being your heart wants to align with in your life for these next forty days that will serve your highest good. It might be "I am love" or "I feel worthy." Many women love the statement "I am enough." If it feels right, you can use just one simple word, like *peace* or *allow*. Ultimately, the intention that's right for you comes in your own words.

You always want to word your intention as if it has already happened because during yoga nidra, intentions imprint in the fertile space of your subconscious mind, where anything you plant can grow. One woman in my program, whose financial situation had radically shifted to a challenging place after the death of her partner so that she needed to increase her business revenue, shared with me that she was repeating the primary intention "I am readying myself to be of service" during her daily yoga nidra. Gently, I pointed out that her intention was not phrased as though it were already true right now, and I suggested that if it felt right, she might want to change it to "I am of service." She liked my suggestion, but she put it into her own language and included a reference to her health, which had suffered since her partner's death. Her intention became "I am in rhythm with my body, sleep, and creativity." Two months later, she was beginning to see signs of her vibrant self, and she had finished her new website. While we do not use the intention to produce an outcome, the pompom-shaking truth is that aligning with your intention often sets in motion the wheels that move you toward reaching specific goals.

Typically, when women go through the three-step process of discovering their intention, they find one they like. But occasionally, someone won't. If this is you, I suggest you use the intention "I am a well-rested woman" during phase one, or practice without an intention and let one come to you while practicing yoga nidra meditation. Intentions often arise spontaneously when you're asked to state your intention during a yoga nidra meditation. Be patient and let the right intention come to you in its own time.

Also don't get hung up on getting your intention right or perfect. (Remember our Daring to Rest mantra: chuck perfect.) Many times, when you think you have a great intention, you might feel inspired to tweak it after a new soul whisper arises during a later yoga nidra session. As you continue to practice your yoga nidra meditations in the days ahead, don't be afraid to adjust your intention statement if you get a soul whisper that deeply resonates in your heart.

Use your new intention for the first time during your day 6 yoga nidra meditation, presented in the next chapter.

Your Intention Continues Working on Your Behalf

After a while, when you wake from yoga nidra, your intention will be programmed into your entire being, so the moment you stray off your intention, you'll feel it, and your subconscious will naturally redirect you back to your intention. That means you don't have to do anything to accomplish this intention.

This scenario happens all the time with the women I coach. Margreet came from a dynamic of not feeling safe with her emotionally needy mother, and this paralyzed her in many areas of her adult life. She had tried talk therapy, and while it was helpful, she never felt a deep shift in her issues of safety until she began practicing yoga nidra.

Her intention was simple, but powerful: "I am safe." Very quickly, she felt this truth in her body and with her children. The more she felt safe, the more she gained confidence, and her exhausting dynamic with her mother began to improve as she developed a new perspective. Today, as a result of feeling safe for the first time in her adult life, she is not running herself to exhaustion, but instead, through aligning in her yoga nidra meditation with the feeling of her intention, she is finally free from the chains of her childhood story with her mother.

When an intention imprints into your subconscious mind, there is a profound shift in priorities. You take action as if it's your mission in life, but this action is not fueled by "doing" at any cost. Margreet has her yoga nidra practice, and this grounds her back to her intention and, at the same time, deeply relaxes her body, so she is able to manage physical exhaustion. On the days when she feels those old safety issues rise she tells me she will often practice yoga nidra twice, to keep her internal power switch fully on and to stay connected to her intention.

I get asked all the time, "When will I start to see my intention take hold in my life?" This is a normal question given how our culture trains us to want results for effort. What you have to remember is that an intention is not being planted to do anything more than point you back to your most authentic self and purpose in life. How the intention expresses itself in your life may be obvious quickly, but it varies from person to person. And sometimes we don't see specific tangible results, like a new job, but rather changes in our state of mind that often lead to getting a new job. You may feel more vibrant or less worried. For Margreet, feeling safe did not suddenly mean she had lots of contact with her mother. Instead, she came to a more peaceful place in their relationship.

There isn't a checklist to tell you when your intention has taken hold; that's not the point of yoga nidra. You practice with your intention until you feel ready for a new one or until a new one presents itself during your yoga nidra meditation. Without an attachment to an end result, you are truly free to just rest. I always tell women, "You don't have to work on yoga nidra. Let it work on you." The same goes for intention. During these first five days, let the focus be on rest and listening to your soul whispers without a huge investment in getting the *right* intention for the next forty days. Your intention will come.

Optional: Diving Deeper

Looking to dive more deeply into your intentions, soul whispers, and rest? Consider these Daring to Rest optional prompts:

- Freewrite in a journal about your soul whispers. Instructions on how to freewrite can be found in chapter three.

- If your intention were a dance, how would it move? Dance your intention.

- Paint or draw a tree with your intention as the tree trunk and your soul whispers above the tree, as clouds in the sky, or below the tree, as roots.

- What activities take priority for you over rest? Which ones could you shift so you can find time to rest? Do you ever purposely avoid rest? If so, why? Freewrite to reflect on these questions.

Key Points in Chapter Four

- Setting an intention is an important part of yoga nidra meditation.

- Your intention should be a positive statement that captures what your heart desires, but not based on outcome. You'll use this intention throughout the Rest phase, with the option to change it when you enter the Release and Rise phases.

- The "Discovering Your Intention" process helps you find one to three words from your soul whispers that resonate deeply with you. You can then add "I," "I am," or "I feel" in front of these words to form your intention. You may need to tweak your intention statement to find one that resonates for you, but always use your soul whisper words in your intention statement.

- Soul whisper words that feel negative can be changed into positive words to create an intention by noting what the opposite word would be.

- If you receive nothing as a soul whisper on any day, or if you don't receive any words for your intention, that's okay. Let your intention come to you later, or start with "I am a well-rested woman" as your intention.

5

BODY

Feeling Grounded,
Relaxed, and Safe

Days 6-10

Your best teacher is your physical body. Rarely does illness or burnout happen without warning, and normally the first clues we get are in our physical bodies. But most of us aren't listening, right? Well, now is your time to pay attention to your body. Yoga nidra invites you to deeply relax your entire body and safely feel again.

For the next five days, all I want you to do is practice yoga nidra, notice how relaxed you feel, and when you are not practicing yoga nidra, begin to sense when you feel grounded and when you don't. The focus of these five days is cleaning the physical body. Of the five bodies of awareness, your physical body is the most dense and solid. The other four bodies are energy states; you can sense but not see them. Connecting to your physical body helps you surrender to rest, relax deeply, and check how grounded you feel in your life.

Basic Instructions for Days 6 to 10

1. Practice the Phase One: Rest Meditation daily. Use the intention you received after your first five days and hold your touchstone in your left hand or place it at the base of your spine, between your legs, near your perineum.

2. Continue to listen for and track your soul whispers in a journal.

3. Optional: Use additional practices to balance your physical body.

4. Optional: Use prompts to help you dive deeper into your soul whispers and issues of safety and groundedness.

Feeling Safe in Your Body Again

Our physical bodies hold struggles with our existence: Do I belong on this earth? Is it safe for me to be here? Safety and fear are concerns of your first power center. If a woman doesn't say yes to her existence, her body will express her no or her doubts as health issues or fatigue. When you have a basic trust in life and lack of fear, your physical body thrives. When you don't, you tend to feel worn out.

When women initially come to me, they are often feeling ungrounded in their lives. Relaxing deeply is key to feeling grounded again. When you lie down in your yoga nidra meditation for the next five days, notice how it feels to be so close to the ground. It doesn't matter if you're not literally on the ground but instead practicing on a bed, in a chair, or on a building's upper floor. By guiding you to rotate your attention through your body and breathe in specific ways, yoga nidra helps you feel present in your body, relaxed, and connected to the earth.

Whatever you feel as you practice yoga nidra, try not to judge it. For some women, it simply feels deeply nourishing to lie down and relax. But if you've been in survival mode for a long time, lying down and feeling your body may be initially uncomfortable. That's okay—let yoga nidra be your umbilical cord back to feeling. Let it help you bless and then leave behind discomfort, broken feelings, or perhaps pain, and find your way back to health and safety. This is the theme of these next five days.

Silence facilitates safety, if we allow it to, and silence is a key feature of yoga nidra. There's so much noise in our everyday lives, but when you begin practicing yoga nidra, you enter what a woman in my rest program called "the garden of silence." This silence is like a whisper giving you permission to feel your body again. You may not have experienced silence for a long time. I found silence to be the first thing about yoga nidra that made it feel so yummy because, as a mom, I rarely experienced silence. For others, silence may initially feel uncomfortable, but stick with it. Silence is the key to entering your inner world, where you know you are always safe and welcomed.

But yoga nidra goes much deeper than silence. Margreet, whom you met in chapter four, felt this pretty quickly. "I didn't know there was more than just silence," she said. "If you miss affection from a parent, you're always trying to keep busy, never really receiving such deep silence." Suddenly, with yoga nidra, Margreet's body began to release years of tension. "I realized this deep silence gave me the level of safety I needed to truly relax."

Rotating attention through the physical body, the first step in a yoga nidra practice, begins to guide you out of the survival spin mode. When we're in this mode, our adrenals pump cortisol and adrenaline nonstop, which wears out the body. Margreet was stuck in this pattern for years, until she began practicing yoga nidra. As she said, "I was a dry river, and now there's water in the riverbed." Our yoga nidra meditation starts with sensing the physical body, because doing that opens the door to our life-sustaining river of energy, allowing it to flow again into our dry riverbeds.

It can be challenging to fill your riverbed when you've been dry for many years. Aditi, who had experienced two ectopic pregnancies—one of which almost took her life—eventually gave birth to a baby girl. But during the pregnancy, she was filled with fear that the baby would be stillborn, and her birth experience was traumatic. Eventually, she went on anti-anxiety medication. Soon after, she discovered yoga nidra meditation. While she found it deeply relaxing, it was uncomfortable for her to focus on her body without judgment. After all she had been through, she distrusted her body. But she stuck with it, and very soon the body sensing was exactly what helped her trust her body again. She felt water returning to her riverbed.

As she explained, "Each time I would sense another body part, and while it wasn't comfortable, I would just stay very present to feeling—not just the story that my body had failed me, but what it felt like. I had to notice the darkness. I realized that all the anxiety was because of not noticing. The moment I truly noticed my body, I felt a shift at a cellular level to trusting my body again." While the anti-anxiety pills had helped her, practicing yoga nidra showed her that she still had to do other work. She shared, "Now yoga nidra is my anti-anxiety pill. Now I don't go down the spiraling rabbit hole of disliking my body. The simple body rotation [rotating attention through the physical body] gave me the permission to stop stuffing anything. And this was my ticket to freedom."

As you practice yoga nidra meditation daily, I'd like you to notice how free you feel. Maybe it's free from tension or pain. Maybe it's freedom from your to-do list. Freedom looks different for everyone, but freedom, safety, and a good life have an intimate bond. I often think of Harriet Tubman, the nineteenth-century civil rights leader in the United States, who led hundreds of slaves to freedom. Why was she leading them to freedom? So they could feel safe. Safety would give them better lives and the opportunity to not just survive, but also thrive. It would restore the water to their riverbeds.

This is what turning on your internal power switch is all about, and it starts in the physical body. So for these five days, focus on noticing feelings in your body and welcoming them all during your yoga nidra practice. This is the first step to changing a paradigm. The worn-out woman pushes feelings away, going into numb mode because it feels like nonstop busy mode gives her no other choice.

The well-rested woman flips this model by making a conscious decision to rest deeply and welcome feelings. This creates a sense of groundedness and safety. You can shift out of anxiety and so much more, but you've got to be committed to a new paradigm. Yoga nidra helps you easily lie down and do that. In addition, during the next five days, you can try any of the following practices to continue welcoming sensations and balancing your physical body outside of your yoga nidra practice.

Optional: Additional Practices for Your Physical Body

While fifteen minutes of yoga nidra is all you need to do for days 6 through 10, there are additional simple ways to balance your physical body. Following are some of my favorites.

Activate the First Power Center

Your physical body represents safety and so does the first power center. As you already know, the Phase One: Rest Meditation guides you to activate this center. During your yoga nidra practice, you may wish to put your touchstone at your perineum, the part of your body that houses the first power center, to invite feelings of safety and security.

In addition to practicing yoga nidra, you can activate the first power center in other ways. You can put a few drops of a calming essential oil, such as lavender or chamomile, on your clothes every day. Or after practicing yoga nidra, put a drop on the palm of your hands, rub your hands together, bring them to your nose, and then inhale four times. Note that essential oils are not recommended for use during pregnancy unless under the supervision of an experienced aromatherapist. Please check the safety of all essential oils before use and be sure they're mixed in a neutral carrier oil like organic jojoba or almond oil before you apply them to your skin. Undiluted essential oils should not be applied directly to your skin.

Wearing red clothing will also activate the first power center.

Anointing Practice for the Rest Phase

To help you slow down, come back to center, and reconnect with yourself and the earth, you may want to add this beautiful essential oil practice at the end of your yoga nidra meditations during the Rest phase (through day 15). This practice was created by master essential oil blender and energy medicine healer Deborah Sullivan for an online course we co-taught called The Power of Yoga Nidra and Essential Oils. You can read the following instructions slowly into a recording device.

Sit or lie down in a comfortable position and focus on the breath, taking a couple of deep sighs. Place a few drops of a calming essential oil, like lavender or chamomile, on the palms of your hands. Gently massage your palms together, warming and releasing the aroma.

Bring your palms to your nose and take four deep, full breaths. Move your head side to side to breathe through both nostrils. As you feel the scent envelop you, imagine yourself realigning, being restored, and coming into balance with the heavens and the earth. Anoint your forehead, heart, and feet with your essential oil.

As you continue to breathe in the scent, bring your awareness to the space above you. Draw the energy from the heavens down into your crown, forehead, body, and subtle bodies. Feel the scent falling down and showering you with golden, luminous light from the heavens.

Now bring your attention to the space below your body and feet. Feel the beautiful energy of the earth rising up into your feet, legs, and torso, blessing you as it does.

Now feel the energy of the earth and the golden, luminous light of the heavens merging at the heart. You are drawing the heavens from above and the earth from below into your heart.

Feel the balance between the heavens and the earth rippling out from your heart, into your energy field above your head, below your feet, to the left, to the

right, behind, and in front of you. Feel cocooned in
this light and surrounded by the scent anchoring you,
between the heavens and the earth, in your heart.

Move your hands and bless yourself and Mother
Earth in each of the four directions (south, west, north,
east) and then above, below, and within at your heart.
Now bring your hands down to the earth to offer your
blessings to our Mother Earth and all your relations.

Lie on the Ground

One of the best ways to increase support for your physical system is
to lie on the ground outside, in Mother Nature. You can do this for
just five or ten minutes. If your shoulders are tight, put a small pillow
underneath them to let yourself fully surrender. Or practice your fifteen
minutes of yoga nidra outside. Grounding to the earth reduces inflammation in the body, which can help autoimmune and allergic responses
and soothe swollen joints. It can also calm fears and boost your mood.

Sixty-One-Point Relaxation

There is a beautiful sixty-one-point relaxation practice that is sometimes
used during yoga nidra but can also be used on its own. In fact, you'll
recognize it from the Phase One: Rest Meditation that you've already
been using and can use the guidance in appendix 1 for reading it into
a recording device. It's a great way to quickly release tension from the
body at any time during the day or when you go to bed at night.

During the sixty-one-point relaxation, attention is rotated around
the body to *marma* points, areas in the body where life-force energy is
concentrated. These points are often located at the meeting point of two
or more tissues, like muscles, bones, or joints. By rotating attention to
each marma point, you are cleaning blocked energy from the body.

Following are the sixty-one points. It's important to rotate your
attention on each point in the order listed (although, you should not
say or think the numbers when bringing your attention to the point).

1. Point between the eyebrows

2. Hollow of the throat

3. Right shoulder joint

4. Right elbow joint

5. The bend of the right wrist joint

6. Tip of the right thumb

7. Tip of the right index finger

8. Tip of the right middle finger

9. Tip of the right fourth finger (ring finger)

10. Tip of the right small finger

11. The bend of the right wrist joint

12. Right elbow joint

13. Right shoulder joint

14. Hollow of the throat

15. Left shoulder joint

16. Left elbow joint

17. The bend of the left wrist joint

18. Tip of the left thumb

19. Tip of the left index finger

20. Tip of the left middle finger

21. Tip of the left fourth finger (ring finger)

22. Tip of the left small finger

23. The bend of the left wrist joint

24. Left elbow joint

25. Left shoulder joint

26. Hollow of the throat

27. Heart center

28. Right nipple

29. Heart center

30. Left nipple

31. Heart center

32. Solar plexus (just below the bottom of the chest bone)

33. Navel center (two inches below the physical navel)

34. Right hip joint

35. Right knee joint

36. Right ankle joint

37. Tip of the right big toe

38. Tip of the right second toe

39. Tip of the right third toe

40. Tip of the right fourth toe

41. Tip of the right small toe

42. Right ankle joint

43. Right knee joint

44. Right hip joint

45. Navel center (two inches below the physical navel)

46. Left hip joint

47. Left knee joint

48. Left ankle joint

49. Tip of the left big toe

50. Tip of the left second toe

51. Tip of the left third toe

52. Tip of the left fourth toe

53. Tip of the left small toe

54. Left ankle joint

55. Left knee joint

56. Left hip joint

57. Navel center (two inches below the physical navel)

58. Solar plexus (just below the bottom of the chest bone)

59. Heart center

60. Hollow of the throat

61. Point between the eyebrows

When rotating your attention throughout the points, you want to be sure to not visualize each part of your body, which is tempting. Body sensing is more about experiencing how that point *feels*, rather than seeing it clearly in your mind's eye. It may be helpful to visualize a blue dot landing on each marma point or to imagine blocked energy releasing from that point.

Mindful Movement

It can be useful to prepare for yoga nidra by doing ten to fifteen minutes of slow, mindful movement beforehand. This type of movement activates your energy body, and you'll more easily release tension and energy blockages as you rotate your attention through the physical body during your yoga nidra meditation. Here are a few mindful movement suggestions:

- Practice yin yoga, a type of yoga in which you hold the poses for longer periods of time.

- Go on a labyrinth walk.

- Practice walking meditation. To do this, walk slowly
  and, as Buddhist monk and peace activist Thich
  Nhat Hanh says, let your feet kiss the earth.

- Practice tai chi or qigong.

- Move to an instrumental song that has a slow beat.
  The music of the late Gabrielle Roth is excellent for this
  purpose, but you may have other music that you like.

Open Your Feminine Highway

Sensing so many women's lack of intimacy with and acceptance of
their female body and feminine essence, I asked my longtime healer,
David Wright, how women can become more open to radiant health
and healing. His answer was simple: open the feminine highway.

Your feminine highway begins in the physical body at the base of
your spine. It's here, for women, that the soul is anchored and drawn
down into the physical realm. Without this anchor, we don't feel safe
on earth. And that's when the not feeling worthy or loved tapes start
playing, big time.

Women have a long history of rejecting their womanhood due to
cultural expectations that see feminine energy as weakness. In many
ways, through models that sexualize women and girls, laws that hold
women back from leadership, and childbirth practices that silence
mothers' voices, we've been raised to be at war with our feminine
nature and, by extension, ourselves. Consequently, the more we fear
our power as a woman, the harder it becomes to access our feminine
energy, the part of us that is intuitive, creative, and receptive. When
this feminine energy becomes blocked, we view the world only through
a masculine-energy lens of logic and striving. We forget to feel, and we
become angry with ourselves for showing emotion.

As a result, too many women today are leading with only masculine energy, pressured to rush and not nurture or to be busy and
not calm, which puts them into the all-too-familiar worn-out woman

mode. Masculine energy without feminine energy is incomplete, and as a consequence, you don't feel whole.

Please be aware that women as well as men have both masculine and feminine energy, so this is not just about gender. It's about *how* women lead, not whether we are capable of leading. It's about being a woman who *feels*, not thinks, she matters.

What's so beautiful about yoga nidra is that it teaches you to unblock all your energy, including your feminine energy, which helps you lead from a consistently balanced place. This exercise to open your feminine highway is a way to unblock your feminine energy without practicing yoga nidra meditation. You'll feel you can take whatever comes at you in life and transform it because you have access to both your feminine and masculine energies.

When David taught this exercise in one of my yoga nidra programs, everyone loved it. It can be practiced right before or after yoga nidra meditation, or really at any time, even while you're watching television. The results are incredible. One women told me, "All the feelings around my pain as a burden were released." Even if you have experienced sexual trauma, this exercise is safe because putting your hands on yourself puts you in control. If you are in active trauma, you will want to check with your care provider before doing this exercise, but for most women, it is a beautiful way to help you feel safe and powerful in your body.

Here is how you open your feminine highway:

1. Think of your hands as electrodes. Place your right hand on your perineum, the space below your vagina.

2. Lay your left hand over the center of your chest, putting the center of your hand over your breast plate.

3. Hold your hands there for about five minutes. Relax and be as comfortable as you can. You don't need to be thinking about anything special.

Optional: Diving Deeper

Looking to dive more deeply into your soul whispers and issues of safety and groundedness? Consider these Daring to Rest optional prompts:

- Freewrite about the following: Where in your body do you feel safe, and where don't you feel safe? What does safety look like for you in your life?

- Turn on instrumental drumming music and move to the statement "I feel grounded" for one song. After you stop, describe the feeling in your body. Can you say even more about how you feel?

- Draw, paint, or freewrite your soul whispers. Is there a predominant theme? If so, what?

Key Points in Chapter Five

- The physical body is the first of the five bodies of awareness. When we are grounded in our physical bodies, we feel relaxed and safe.

- Rotating attention through the physical body, the first step in a yoga nidra practice, begins to guide you out of the survival spin mode.

- Noticing sensation in your physical body opens the door to a flow of life-sustaining energy and helps you trust your body again.

- Freedom, safety, and a good life have an intimate bond. The more you practice yoga nidra, the more safe and free you will feel.

6

ENERGY

Welcoming Back Your Life Force

Days 11–15

n a yoga nidra meditation, we start with putting our attention on the physical body, and then we bring it to the energy body, normally in the form of conscious breathing, or breath work, because this type of breathing helps move *prana*, or life force. If you're worn out, you're often starved of life force, an energy running through you that gives you vitality. When you practice breath work, you're impacting the energy body, unblocking channels in the body where life force is stuck. The more energy flows in your body, the better your body begins to feel, and often health issues start to improve. Balancing one of the five bodies helps the others, and balancing all of the bodies of awareness can take you back to wholeness.

Many times a yoga nidra meditation makes reference to connecting to your life force or asks you to take a slow, deep breath in and out because breath helps you connect to your life force, and this begins to calm the body. For anyone suffering from anxiety, taking slow, deep breaths that shift your life force to a calmer place can be life changing. A racing heart rate will slow with conscious breathing. Palms and forehead will go back to normal temperature, and slowly, a feeling of ease in both body and mind will return. The energy body does not ask us to try very hard to achieve this feeling of ease. In fact, the opposite is true: these next five days are about continuing to rest deeply with yoga nidra and not trying to make it a perfect experience. Let conscious breath work during yoga nidra give the energy body permission to release all blocked areas and restore your life force.

Basic Instructions for Days 11 to 15

1. Practice the Phase One: Rest Meditation daily. Continue to use the intention you used for days 6 through 10, but feel free to tweak your intention if inspired during your yoga nidra meditation or through your soul whispers. Also continue to keep your touchstone with you when practicing, either in your left hand or placed in the second power center area, anywhere above the pubic bone and below the navel.

2. Continue to listen for and track your soul whispers in a journal.

3. Optional: Use additional practices to support the balance of your energy body.

4. Optional: Use prompts to dive deeper into this chapter's concepts—vitality, slowing down, and rhythm.

Conscious Breath Work

When you breathe consciously during yoga nidra, or any intentional breath work, you are impacting the energy body and unblocking your life force.

Your nostrils are connected to your autonomic nervous system through the neuromotor system in your body. The neuromotor responses influence the brain and activate chemicals, which means whatever nostril you breathe through determines what energy is activated and what chemicals are released. Breathing in through the right nostril influences the thalamus and hypothalamus glands. Breathing in through the left nostril influences the pituitary gland and hypothalamus. Breathing through both nostrils equally activates your life force. But rarely do we breathe through both nostrils. You may think you do, but if you held a mirror close to your nostrils to see the flow of your breath, you'd find that both nostrils are hardly ever activated at the same time. The way you activate both nostrils is through conscious breath work, which is what you are guided to do every time you lie down to practice yoga nidra meditation.

Conscious breath work creates a link between the physical body and the mind via the energy body. By relaxing the physical body, by means of rotating attention through it, and then balancing the energy body through conscious breathing, we begin to access the third body, where we clear the mind. We'll get to the mind in chapter seven, but for now, the point you need to know is that the breath is the key to the interaction between the body and mind. Our breath keeps our organs healthy, and the way we breathe affects their state. Just think of how a short burst of panicked breathing, like what happens during an anxiety attack, affects the physical body.

Many people don't breathe fully; they hold back the breath and have been doing so their whole lives. I see this all the time in the women I support, and I too spent years not breathing fully. The problem with this is that despite the brain's small size relative to the body, it needs a minimum of 20 percent of the body's oxygen to feel nourished.[1] If you're not taking full, deep breaths and exercising regularly, it's hard to get enough oxygen into your body, and as a consequence, your brain functions less optimally, putting your entire body under stress. Conscious breath work can reverse this stress, awaken vitality, and essentially reboot your entire system.

Conscious breath work practiced during yoga nidra can also help you tap into a deep meditative state, which clears away old patterns, thoughts, and emotions and shifts you into alignment with your most authentic self. As you work with the breath consciously, you awaken the energy body, heightening the potential for healing and transformation. Think of breath work as the fuel that helps your body, mind, and spirit operate with ease. The more you feed yourself with breath work, the more ease you feel. If you don't feed yourself this fuel, you won't run optimally.

Reclaiming Your Vitality

It's a pretty simple equation: unblocking energy in your body activates life force, and your vitality begins to return. The problem is, most worn-out women have gotten so used to living with a lack of vitality that it has become their baseline. What happens when we live with less vitality? We get triggered easily by situations and feel uncentered, and for many women, panic attacks, depression, and sleep issues start to appear. Breath work increases life force, which impacts your level of vitality.

During these next five days, as you practice yoga nidra, notice how your vitality shifts from when you begin a yoga nidra meditation to the time you end it. Many women report feeling stressed when they begin yoga nidra, and then by the end, they feel as if they're being cradled or as if their vitality has shifted to a better place. Breath work plays a major role in creating this sense of deep relaxation because it releases blocked life force. As a result, women feel more energetic and awake in the areas of their lives that have been starved of vitality.

Your sex life and intimacy with others is one life area that is often dramatically affected by a lack of vitality. Liz, a woman in her sixties, had felt a sense of inadequacy in her relationship for over four decades. When she began to practice yoga nidra, her first soul whisper was, "Give it up." On the second day, it was, "I am." On the third day, she had an unexpected surprise. Just before listening for her soul whisper, when prompted at the end of yoga nidra to send light to an area of her body that needed healing, the light went to her genitals. "This is embarrassing," she shared, "but I had an orgasm." While having an orgasm isn't common in yoga nidra, it can happen, because yoga nidra activates life force, and as a result, often your vitality returns in all areas of your body.

Liz decided to write down "sex" as her soul whisper for that third day. Then on day 4, she got "contentment." On the fifth day, when she read her soul whispers, they said, "Give it up I am sex contentment." She couldn't believe what she was reading. She shared with the women in our rest program, "I have held inside me for forty-five years a deep resentment toward my husband for things that happened at the beginning of our marriage having to do with sex. As a result, I have been punishing him at the detriment of my own pleasure. It is something I have held onto for so long. This string of words spelled it out for me. 'Give it up.' 'I am' worthy of pleasure. 'Sex' is pleasure. I will be 'content.'" Through yoga nidra, Liz's life force was activated, and listening to her soul whispers made this clear to her. Awareness is the first step to creating change, whether it's a better marriage or needing to end a marriage.

Liz's experience makes sense because yoga nidra releases the energy pools coiled up in the pelvis. In tantra philosophy, this energy is called "the sleeping snake," or *kundalini*. If you've lost touch with your sexual self, experienced abuse, or are just not breathing deeply, then you may have a harder time accessing this sexual energy. But it's there, and you can activate it through the practice of yoga nidra meditation. Be patient. When you combine this practice with listening to your soul whispers, there's great potential for healing any kind of shame and activating vitality.

Life force is the fuel that helps increase our vitality and give birth to anything—a baby, a book, a business. When you're full of vitality, you feel you can do anything. You feel fully alive. Liz's message reminded her that she was worthy of feeling fully alive. Please don't hold back for forty-five years like she did. Listening for your soul whispers during yoga nidra meditation, and looking closely at them afterward to discern their messages, will give you a clear indication of just how fully alive you feel. Soul whispers are like a vitality barometer. They always point out what's not working and point us back to our most vital self. They are powerful instructions for taking your yoga nidra meditation into your everyday life.

Optional: Additional Practices for Your Energy Body

As you already know, your Phase One: Rest Meditation guides you to activate your energy body with a specific type of breathing. Here are some additional practices to help you balance your energy body.

Activate the Second Power Center

Your energy body is connected to your second power center, which represents vitality, passion, and creativity. This center also governs the area above the pubic bone and below the navel. To activate this power center, you may wish to place your Daring to Rest touchstone anywhere on this area of your body during your yoga nidra meditation during days 11 through 15.

You might also like to use a few drops of mandarin orange essential oil on your clothes or on your hands. Wearing orange clothing will also support the activation of the second power center.

Use Water

Soak in a warm bath or take a warm shower to get creative ideas flowing. Put on drumming music or any transformational dance music to listen to while in the tub or shower.

If you have menstrual cramps, use a hot water bottle in your pelvic area to release unwanted energy in the second power center.

If you live near water, go for a swim and then practice yoga nidra meditation near the water.

Cooling Breath

Also known as *sheetali*, the Cooling Breath relaxes the body and mind. You'll recognize it from the Phase One: Rest Meditation, but it's a great stand-alone breath-work technique to use when you feel anxiety or intense emotions or thoughts. I like to call it "the straw breath," because when you exhale, you purse your lips as if you're blowing through a straw. Here's how to do it:

1. Lie or sit down.

2. Inhale slowly, filling the abdomen, then the chest, and then the chest cavity, all the way up to the neck.

3. Exhale even more slowly, pursing your lips as if you're blowing through a straw.

4. Repeat four to six times—or as many times as you'd like.

5. When you stop, spend a minute tuning in to how the breath has impacted your body. Track how and where you feel this impact.

Alternate Nostril Breathing

Yogis consider alternate nostril breathing one of the best breath-work techniques for calming the mind and nervous system. It also balances the right- and left-brain functions. Start with three rounds in a session. After you feel comfortable with this technique, you can add rounds until you are comfortable doing seven rounds in a session. If you'd like to see this breath demonstrated in a video, there are lots of examples on the Internet. Here are the steps for Alternate Nostril Breathing:

1. Close the right nostril with your right thumb.

2. Inhale through the left nostril for a count of four, or about four seconds.

3. Immediately close the left nostril with your right ring finger and little finger. At the same time, remove your thumb from the right nostril.

4. Exhale through the right nostril for a count of eight, or about eight seconds.

5. Keeping your right ring and little fingers in place, inhale through the right nostril to the count of four.

6. Close the right nostril with your right thumb.

7. Exhale through the left nostril to the count of eight. This completes one full round.

Pay Attention to Rhythm

Rest and rhythm are best friends. Rest looks after rhythm, and rhythm looks after rest. The more you begin to honor rhythm in your life, the easier it will be to tap back into your vitality.

A simple way to become in sync with rhythm during these next five days is to watch the sunset in the evening or the sunrise in the early morning. Watching the sunset is a particularly good idea for people with sleep issues. It sends a message to your body to slow down and start producing melatonin for sleep. If you can't observe the sun setting, you can honor it by turning off the lights in your home at dusk. Light some candles if you want to, or just sit in your home quietly and notice how your home goes from light to dark. This will help your body and mind slow down and connect to your life force.

Beyond these five days, another way to pay attention to rhythm is to chart your menstruation. Note on your calendar or in your Daring to Rest journal when your period starts, and note the blood flow and feelings that come with it. On the first day of your menstruation, look in the mirror and repeat the phrase, "I am fully alive." Don't menstruate? Then note the date of the full moon each month, and on that date, look in the mirror and repeat, "I am fully alive" several times that day.

Rhythm is always happening around us; the key to feeling more peaceful and full of vitality is to notice it and arrange your life to live more aligned with your cycles and rhythms.

Optional: Diving Deeper

Looking to dive more deeply into vitality, slowing down, and rhythm? Consider these Daring to Rest optional prompts:

- Review your five soul whispers from days 11 through 15. If you got an image for your soul whisper, give your image a one-word title. String the words from your soul whispers together to create one sentence. Draw a picture of this sentence or freewrite about this sentence and how it relates to your current vitality.

- What are some ways you could slow down? Freewrite about slowing down.

- If your body were a song, what would it be called and how would it move? Express the rhythm in your body through movement.

- Freewrite in a journal about your soul whispers.

- Describe your experience of yoga nidra mediation in one word. Using this word as a starting point, freewrite about your experience with yoga nidra meditation.

Key Points in Chapter Six

- Your energy body is the second of five bodies of awareness.

- During yoga nidra, breath work (conscious breathing) balances the energy body and unblocks your life force. As a result, you feel more vitality, passion, and creativity.

- Life force is the fuel that helps increase our vitality, and this helps us give birth to anything—a baby, a book, a business.

- Your soul whispers hold clues to your level of vitality.

Phase Two

RELEASE

Whatever you meet, you can go beyond.

For the next fifteen days you'll be clearing the second layer of exhaustion: emotional and mental exhaustion. Yoga nidra meditation does this effortlessly every time you lie down to practice, but for fifteen days we'll be exploring these layers more deeply. This is the huge unexpected benefit of yoga nidra: you are getting deep rest and being pointed back to your internal power switch, which is like sleep and good therapy in one—and with quicker results. But before you begin day 16 of your Daring to Rest journey, I want to introduce you to a theme that captures yoga nidra's magic: making friends with darkness.

There's a beautiful Marianne Williamson quote that says, "Until we have seen someone's darkness, we don't really know who that person is."[1] During this second phase, I'll be asking you to meet and greet the dark sides of yourself. Meeting your darkness is a key to feeling powerful. Practicing yoga nidra meditation encourages you to engage with difficult emotions and beliefs because darkness can help you find your way home to your internal power switch. The more you avoid meeting darkness, the harder it will be to feel calm and peaceful.

Have you ever noticed how our culture demonizes the dark, and how darkness has virtually disappeared at night? Light pollution is everywhere. The consequences of our disdain for night, and the effects of overexposure to light, are now appearing in many places on our planet. Sleep disorders are skyrocketing. Night light is confusing bird migratory patterns. The twenty-four-hour day-night cycle, known as the circadian clock, affects everything from hormone production to cell regulation. When you disrupt your circadian clock, you are at a higher risk for medical issues including depression, insomnia, cardio-vascular disease, and cancer. The body produces melatonin at night, but if you're exposed to light, then melatonin levels drop. Studies are finding that decreased melatonin levels lead to an increase in your risk for cancer. In fact, night-shift workers, like nurses, who are exposed to indoor light at night are showing increased rates for breast cancer.[2] Even sleeping with a night-light on has shown a small but measurable increase in the risk for breast cancer in women.

Mythology also holds clues on the importance of night. The Greek goddess of night, Nyx, had many children, and one was Hypnos, the god of sleep. Yes, in Greek mythology, *sleep is the child of night.* This is ironic given all the sleep problems in the world. Nyx was mar-ried to her brother, Erebus, the god of depth and darkness, and they also gave birth to Hypnos's twin brother, Thanatos, the god of death. No wonder we fear going to sleep: night and darkness bring death. This message is ingrained in us from an early age: we should be afraid of the dark because darkness means danger. Many of us feel this in our psyche. As children, we expressed it to our parents as, "I'm afraid there are monsters in my room." As adults, we shove this belief into a pocket of our unconscious mind, but that doesn't extinguish it. Yoga nidra asks us to engage with these thoughts instead of distancing ourselves from them. To darkness, it would say, "Come closer."

With yoga nidra, we begin to see the possibility of meeting dark-ness and, by extension, embracing the night. Nyx's children weren't all death and doom. She also had a daughter, Elpis, the goddess of hope. *Hope is also the child of night.* This is so true with any breakthrough: if you can just hang on through it, meeting all your dark emotions and thoughts, you will break through. You'll enter midnight, the darkest moment, and it's here you'll welcome everything just as it is, both dark and light. This is when grace arrives. You will feel it filling you—a holy presence, a stillness in your heart, a peace that permeates your entire being. Joy arrives, ego drops away, and your fearful sense of self falls away. Every time you lie down to practice yoga nidra, you're being safely led into this dance with your shadowy sides.

The moment you say yes to meeting your darkness, something incredible happens: you start breaking the cycle of fatigue. Why? Because often a dark emotion just wanted a little attention, and once it gets your attention, its power diffuses. You begin to feel more at ease. I know it's hard to take the first step, but yoga nidra guides you there gently and effortlessly. It may seem counterintuitive to think that meeting a dark emotion or thought would make you feel better, but your attention to darkness is ultimately your ticket to less exhaustion.

Occasionally, there's a woman who enrolls in one of my yoga nidra programs with the intention to meet her darkness. Deborah, who entered my Daring to Rest program having suddenly lost her partner of sixteen and a half years, fit this category: intelligent, spiritual, having years of experience guiding women through spiritual journeys, and eager to meet the darkness she felt so deeply.

When Deborah started the rest immersion program, she was shattered at the sudden loss of her beloved, a man she knew was her soul mate from the moment she met him. His death reorganized her entire world. For the first few months after his death, she had support from others, but after that, she felt that she had to put on a mask for people she couldn't show her grief to. She tried going to a grief counselor but quickly knew that she couldn't think or talk her way out of grief.

Yoga nidra became her "unconditional mother," her safe space to meet herself, meet all her darkness and the light, and greet transformation. "It met me exactly where I was," she said. During yoga nidra meditation, she could see how grief was showing up in her body and systems. Deborah shares, "It was such a mirroring of what was going on inside of me, what in the external world I had no words for yet." Until practicing yoga nidra, she had no idea how deeply her grief was living in her cells.

"Yoga nidra is like the alchemist's caldron," she explained. "It was a place that I could garden and harvest everything within me that is beautiful and not beautiful."

Yoga nidra didn't ask Deborah to not grieve. Her darkness was held in love, and then in that holding, she realized that she could go on without her beloved partner. She could embrace the darkness and choose not to let it consume her.

In phase two, you will have this same opportunity to work with any darkness you're holding. Grief can come from any form of loss—losing a beloved family member, losing a job you loved, leaving a community of friends, or moving away from a location you loved. When we lose something, we often fall into a place of feeling broken. And this broken feeling disconnects us from our internal power switch. A woman disconnected from her internal power switch feels weak and unsure, and this opens her to voices that say, "I'm worthless," or "I'm fat," or in Deborah's case, "I'm not strong enough to go on after this loss." It's a voice telling you negative or frightening things, further disconnecting you from your confidence.

This voice and its energy can make it very hard to get out of a dark place or to practice self-love, self-care, and self-compassion. This is why it's important to practice yoga nidra often whenever we are feeling overwhelmed by darkness, whether it's grief or some other dark feeling. When you greet dark emotions and really feel them, you are reconnected to your instinct. The voice of fear and negativity cannot penetrate this connection, and as a result, you will not blindly follow it. The moment you make this reconnection, you have begun to turn your internal power switch on. You're effectively saying, "I know I'm not only darkness. That is just a part of me at this moment." This is how you take back darkness, how you embrace the night, and ultimately how you shift out of a dark place to wholeness to embrace your power.

Here in phase two, yoga nidra will help you explore what emotional exhaustion you need to release to feel powerful again. As you move through the next three chapters, it's time to dare to rest on an even deeper level. The veils are coming off, dear Sister. Fatigue is lifting. Keep lying down to wake up. *You've got this.*

7

MIND

Letting Go of Burdens

Days 16-20

The first five days of phase two focus on the third body of awareness, the mental body. The process of yoga nidra begins with balancing the physical and then the energy body, and this prepares you to enter the mental body, where you begin to loosen all the self-defeating habits you've been attached to for a lifetime. The promise of the mental body is big: is it possible to find peace of mind with your everyday life? The answer is yes, you can, and the yoga nidra pompom-shaking excitement is that you can do it lying down.

The mental body governs your rational, linear, and sequential thought processes. It's the body that starts doing the deep cleaning of the mind. This is your opportunity to get out of the mental spin cycle that leaves so many of us exhausted. The mental body is the most important one to understand because it's here where you use your mind to manipulate your world. When your mental body is well balanced, you'll have rational and logical thoughts, which will then influence your actions and interactions with others in a more positive way. You'll feel powerful. But if your mental body is out of balance, then you'll disconnect from rational thought and the truest version of yourself. Not only can panic befall you if you don't clear the conflict in the mental body, but you can also become consumed by your thoughts and feelings and, as a result, take unkind actions. When our minds are full of judgment, we separate ourselves from others and from the bigger picture of the world. Understanding the mental body and keeping it balanced is crucial to managing suffering and starting to feel powerful.

Let me be clear about what is meant by "mind" in the mental body because it might be different from what you think it is. In yoga nidra "mind" is connected with time, space, and causality. In everyday life, the gap between time, space, and causality seems long, but when you meditate, this gap closes. Sometimes when you are in yoga nidra meditation, the mind can even stop. When this gap closes, you are connected to the cosmic mind. Your individual mind has real needs, but yogic teachings and many other spiritual teachings tell us that we're all part of one cosmic mind. When you're practicing yoga nidra, this is the mind you tap into, and it's where you reconnect to your power.

Basic Instructions for Days 16 to 20

1. Practice the Phase Two: Release Meditation daily for five days. Continue to use the intention you crafted in phase one or create a new intention as you're guided to in this chapter. Your new intention can focus on a habit you'd like to break or an issue, like health, that you'd like to address. Also continue to hold your touchstone in your left hand when practicing or place it on your third power center, your gut, in your digestive area.

2. Listen for and track your soul whispers.

3. Optional: Use additional practices to balance your mental body.

4. Optional: Use prompts to dive deeper into warrior energy, darkness, and holding opposites.

From Disconnected to Powerful

To understand what a profound impact balancing the mental body can have on your life, I want you to meet Mae. When Mae arrived in my Daring to Rest immersion program, she had a history of dealing with an ex-husband who was verbally abusive during their marriage, was an alcoholic and drug addict, and had cheated on her with other women. Not surprisingly, Mae's life read like a panic-attack script: high levels of stress for a long period of time and constant judgment on her life experiences. She told me, "I thought living under stress like this was normal." The results? Mae felt completely disconnected from her life and had consistent anxiety and panic attacks. She managed them with medication for years, mostly antidepressants and sleeping pills. But when I met her, all of her usual medications had stopped working, and every new medication suggested by her doctor didn't seem to work either. "I couldn't get on an elevator," Mae told me. "My heart would race, and I'd be sweating." Everyday life felt like a fight-or-flight situation for Mae.

What Mae experienced was an *amygdala hijacking*, to use the term coined by psychologist Daniel Goleman.[1] Your amygdala comprises two masses of gray matter, located inside each cerebral hemisphere. It is involved with the experiencing of emotions. When you're under extreme stress, the amygdala can hijack, or take over, your rational mind, the higher thinking centers in your neocortex that would normally slow down your responses, causing your body to go straight to a fight-or-flight response. In the short term, you want your amygdala to do this because it helps you run away from immediate danger or manage a crisis. In the long term, you don't want your amygdala overriding these thinking centers because a constant release of adrenaline and cortisol into your system for a long period of time can trigger panic attacks, produce an ideal environment for disease, and create unhealthy assumptions based on a one-sided perception of your life.

I think of an amygdala hijacking as the mental spin cycle for women. Imagine your clothes being washed in a washing machine. In the beginning, they're gently being swished around in the water with soap. This is your rational mind; when something gets dirty, you clean it. Then the spin cycle arrives, and this is the moment when the clothes have got to let go of *all* the dirt, not just the surface dirt. The mental spin cycle can be healthy, unless you resist letting go of your mental dirt. Then it's like the washing machine that's stuck on its spin cycle: your amygdala bypasses your rational mind, you disconnect from your power, and you're in freak-out mode, spinning uncontrollably. *He slept around, and I allowed it. I don't know how to get out of my marriage. My ex is dating a twenty-eight-year-old. I'm too shy. I'm too heavy. I don't want pain. I don't want pain. I don't want pain.* Surprise: you're in deep pain—and whether you get eight hours of sleep or not, this kind of spin cycle pain is exhausting.

A balanced mental body can stop this spin cycle from getting out of control, and during yoga nidra, your mental body is brought into balance as you are continually encouraged to feel all your thoughts and emotions. You'd think this is a recipe for disaster, that you'd feel worse. But actually you feel better because yoga nidra doesn't just leave you feeling your misery; it also invites you to feel the opposite, which helps you disidentify with that miserable emotion or thought and brings your mental body into balance.

The Power of Holding Opposites

A key feature of yoga nidra is feeling opposites. During yoga nidra, you are often asked to hold opposite sensations, like hot and cold. This trains your body to stop identifying with only one-half of a pair of opposing sensations. I cannot emphasize enough how freeing holding opposites can be for you. For many women, like Mae, it transformed years of anxiety quite quickly—seeming like a miracle.

In the Phase Two: Release Meditation, you will notice that you are asked to hold pairs of opposite emotions. First you are invited to remember an experience of feeling disconnection, weakness, and powerlessness; then you are invited to allow opposite feelings to arise; and finally, you are invited to welcome both sets of feelings. This is training your mind to hold opposite feelings, which frees you from overidentifying with a feeling and creating the out-of-control mental spin cycle. While holding opposites is common in yoga nidra, holding opposite feelings and thoughts is a classic feature of iRest yoga nidra, developed by Richard Miller. Just imagine feeling angry and being unable to shift out of that anger—for years. Yoga nidra says that it's okay to feel anger, and it's okay to feel the opposite, gentleness or empathy. Both reside in you. When we only acknowledge one, we get stuck in the mental spin cycle.

In Mae's case, holding opposite feelings meant effectively acknowledging her anxiety and then gently pointing out to herself that she had a peaceful place inside of her too. The moment your mind begins to even slightly disidentify from only thinking that you're a panic-attack-driven mess is your ticket to a better place. It's why I call holding opposites the golden magic of yoga nidra meditation.

We're often so busy living our lives in *either-or*—either I'm powerful or I'm disconnected. Viktor Frankl, a prominent Jewish psychiatrist and neurologist in Vienna whose pregnant wife and parents died in the Holocaust, wrote in his book *Man's Search for Meaning* how he consciously chose to live in the space between either-or. Frankl's mind could have easily lived in misery after experiencing the Holocaust, and who would blame him for thinking, "I've lost everyone. My life has no meaning." But Frankl noticed in the concentration camps that the people who were resilient were those who found meaning despite their horrific situation.[2]

I hear a gazillion times from women that the practice Holding Opposites is their breakthrough tool, both while practicing yoga nidra and in their everyday lives. Why? By holding one feeling and then another and then uniting the two feelings, you receive a visceral understanding of a universal law: that all is one. The mental body always has preferences in your everyday life; it's programmed to have ideas about right and wrong. What we forget is that there is also a space of awareness that never changes. In the space of awareness, everything is okay. Painful and stressful memories are still mediated by the amygdala, but holding opposites helps you to not live in the unconscious habits and patterns that get triggered by pain and stress.

Holding Opposites Practice

Here's how you do the Holding Opposites practice:

1. Feel any big emotion or thought in your body. Really engage all of your senses. You may want to think of a memory to bring the sensation forward, but then let go of the memory and stay with the sensation in your body. Take three slow breaths feeling this emotion or thought.

2. Release that sensation and call up the opposite sensation. Again, really engage your senses and use a memory to bring it forward if you need to. Take three slow breaths.

3. Now call up both sensations and feel them at the same time. This is the space between the opposites. Take three slow breaths.

4. Notice how you feel.

Here are some common emotions and emotion-generating states and their opposites:

Angry/loving

Sad/happy

Pessimistic/optimistic

Hopeless/hopeful

Fearful/brave

Exhausted/rested

Lonely/complete

Holding Opposites is also excellent for specific situations that often trigger strong emotions, such as these:

Menstruation: pain/comfort

Pregnancy and birth: fear/trust

Initially, the Holding Opposites practice may feel hard to do, but keep with it. Eventually, you will feel into the space between. When you practice the Phase Two: Release Meditation you are guided to hold opposites, but many people find it useful to use this technique on its own, when their system feels overwhelmed by an emotion or thought.

Pregnancy, for example, is my favorite time to practice Holding Opposites. If you have been practicing yoga nidra throughout pregnancy, then the Holding Opposites practice will be easy to do during birth. Birth is one of the ultimate moments when a woman feels both "I can't do this" and "I can do this"—two very powerful opposites. Today, this battle between fear and trust in giving birth often ends in a woman siding with fear because, unless she has a room full of midwives or doulas believing she can do it, most hospital birthing rooms aren't filled with "you can do it" cheering. The good news is that when practicing Holding Opposites a woman doesn't need others to believe she can birth a baby—she just needs herself.

Clarissa, a woman having her first birth at forty-two, used the Holding Opposites practice as she neared transition in her birth. She told me, "I was so scared, so I felt that, and then I started consciously welcoming the feeling 'I am not scared,' and it was incredible how fast my body relaxed." When she held both, that's when she said she felt "a deep sense of peace." She repeated this practice for about ten minutes, and then her baby was born. That moment a baby is born is the ultimate holding of opposites. It's when a woman drops the *either-or* and says yes to *both-and*.

The Holding Opposites practice helped Monique, a single mom, transform her relationship with her mother. For years, Monique had been upset with her mother because of the emotional support she didn't get as a child. She was haunted by a scary incident she'd experienced when she was five years old: two boys took her to a secluded place and made her raise her shirt. She got away, but when she told her mother, her mother thought Monique was overreacting. Over the years, Monique continued to stay angry with her mother, and eventually, after years of trying to make her mother see her side, Monique's anger turned to rage. The moment she learned to hold opposites during yoga nidra, she could see for the first time how her mother could have her feelings and Monique could have hers. As a result, finally, the rage toward her mother began to lift.

"I used to feel [the only way] to resolve our situation [was] by me only acknowledging how my mother felt," Monique shared. "Now there's space for my feelings and her feelings. We can feel differently about the situation and it's okay." Holding opposites taught Monique that there isn't a right or wrong way to feel. After practicing yoga nidra for a while, "the issue with my mother became a nonissue," she said. She finally felt at peace with it. "This is why I call yoga nidra meditation magic," Monique explained. "You can feel okay with people you've been in conflict with for years."

Just to be clear, disidentifying from a charged emotion like anger does not mean you numb yourself to it. It means exactly the opposite: you're consciously feeling the emotion and, in doing so, you're becoming unstuck from an exhausting mental loop. You may not be ready to have your mother be a part of your life, but you can come to a more peaceful place within you. This is the first step toward feeling well rested. Monique's mother didn't change, but her mother's behavior no longer consistently sends Monique into a place of emotional exhaustion. Her yoga nidra practice helped, but she also uses the Holding Opposites practice outside of yoga nidra. It's a great tool to use to shift any challenging relationship.

The mental body is all about the element of fire. Fire can be used to destroy or to create, as fire turns matter into energy that can be used to move forward. A balanced mental body transforms "my will," ego-driven fire, into "thy will," a force no longer powered by ego. You do this by using the same principle of meeting anger with awareness.

Anger is a low-level, reptilian-brain neural response that forms for most people before the rational mind has a chance to intervene. It does not want to hang out for long. So the moment you give awareness to your anger, you diffuse its emotional charge. The pompom-shaking beauty of yoga nidra is that you can release the fire burning you up through lying down and without tremendous effort.

Like Monique, being able to hold opposite emotions presented Mae with the opportunity to break out of anxiety. She used to feel like her heart was going to explode from every little thing in her life. "I felt so fragile," she told me. She had pushed every feeling away. But experiencing the holding of opposites through yoga nidra showed her that, as she said, "I don't have to stay in all these stories and the related feelings." She also released herself from years of deep resentment the moment she met her resentment and realized the opposite also resided within her. "Everything in my life softened," she said. "Now I'm able to get my mind quiet. Getting quiet feels like a miracle."

Overcoming Negative Habits and Self-Defeating Mental/Emotional Patterns

How was Mae able to start feeling more powerful? She started to clear her mental body by using the power of opposites to let go of her negative emotions and move into a more positive place. When you're holding emotions that no longer serve you, it feels as if heavy boulders have shown up in your life. You often feel numb, oversensitive, and powerless. But meeting these emotions diffuses their charge, and that's when your power returns. Back to the riverbed analogy, balancing the mental body helps more of the free-flowing river return to your dry riverbed.

Your first fifteen days of yoga nidra has been preparing you for this moment, inviting your body to meet sensations and activate your life force. You're now ready to stop repeating negative mental/emotional patterns and self-defeating habits. For example, if you have struggled with overeating, this habit has made an imprint on your mind. The more you repeat the habit, the stronger the imprint becomes, and the harder it is to do the opposite, which in this case would be to not overeat. When a habit pattern has a deep hold over you and alters your body chemistry, it is an addiction. If this addiction continues, it can alter your personality, and suddenly these imprints begin to feel like your destiny.

In Mae's case, struggling with anxiety had become normal for her, and she felt it would be her life. The good news, as yoga nidra teacher and trainer John Vosler points out, is that yoga nidra is like "Mr. Clean" for all five bodies. In the mental body, by using various techniques to shine awareness on the habit pattern, like pairing of opposites, intention, visualization, and affirmations, yoga nidra helps clean up these imprints that formed. When Mae lay down to practice yoga nidra, its Mr. Clean touch trained her mind to stop supporting the imprint that said she must suffer with anxiety. After daily practice, Mae finally realized that her destiny did not have to be a life of anxiety. We think we must live in darkness when, in fact, there is always a flicker of light in the darkest situation. Yoga nidra helped Mae acknowledge the darkness and find the light.

You can work at changing your negative mental/emotional patterns and self-defeating habits by talking about them in therapy and with other methods. But addressing them during yoga nidra meditation is especially effective because in yoga nidra, you go into the deepest state of meditation, where you can work at the roots of these habits and patterns. Mae told me several times that she had spent years in therapy, deep in her personal story, but it wasn't until yoga nidra that she felt the anxiety, and all her personal stories of hardship, finally lift.

It's easy to think you're a loser if you've got a lot of negative habits and patterns that have turned into imprints, and you keep reinforcing them. But you're not alone—everyone is working out the imprints of their habits and patterns. The key is to not let your habits and patterns drive counterproductive behaviors, but instead to witness them in a detached manner. This is not easily done, but in yoga nidra meditation, when you invite the mind to hold opposite pairs—of emotions, thoughts, or situations—you help to remove the dominant habit and/or pattern from your mind, thus balancing the mental body.

When I met Mae, her self-defeating habits and negative patterns had become deep imprints in her mind. Here's what she told herself over and over again: "My husband was a cheater. My parents were horrible to me. I'm a loser mother." When we overidentify with mental imprints like this, very often we express the imbalance somewhere in our life. For Mae, it was expressed through depression and anxiety. Her mind believed her thoughts. Ego was in full control. As a result, Mae felt broken, often repeating the mantra I hear so many women say: "I am not enough."

If this "I am not enough" mantra, or a similar self-defeating thought, is playing in your ear, instead of running from it, meet it with awareness using the power of opposites. What does this mean? Feel "I am not enough" in your body and then welcome the opposite feeling: that you are enough. It seems simple, but doing this again and again stops you from reinforcing the imprints that are causing you to suffer. It cleans your mind. Meeting emotions, thoughts, and deep imprints of the mind with awareness is yoga nidra's superpower.

Optional: Additional Practices for Your Mental Body

Don't be dismayed if old habits and patterns take time to clear. Most people have to balance and rebalance the mental body to keep it clear. But during these next five days, the Phase Two: Release Meditation will begin to open this portal to clearing your mind. Here are some additional practices you can use to help balance your mental body both while practicing yoga nidra and outside of your yoga nidra meditations.

Activate Your Third Power Center

A balanced mental body helps you feel powerful. It's here you can transform anything that no longer serves you. This is warrior energy. The mental body is associated with the third power center, which is located in the space from your navel to breastbone and particularly in your solar plexus, your digestive area. If you have digestive issues or feel lots of anger, I encourage you to activate this third power center by placing your touchstone on your solar plexus during yoga nidra meditation. Blocked energy here is often due to the challenge of digesting one's personal power. You might also like to put a few drops of lemon essential oil on your clothes, or put a drop on the palm of your hands, rub your hands together, and inhale the scent from your hands. Wearing yellow also helps activate the third power center.

Anointing Practice for the Release Phase

This is another beautiful essential oil practice created by Deborah Sullivan that you can add to your yoga nidra meditation for the entire Release phase (days 16 to 30).

Choose any essential oil that is purifying, such as citrus or cypress. Apply a drop to your heart and to any part of your body that is releasing stories, scripts, emotions, and behaviors that don't serve who you are remembering yourself to be.

You may wish to read the following words into a recording device.

> Feel the scent showering you, cleansing, opening, and creating flow in any areas where your energy feels blocked, stagnant, or stuck. Envision the scent infusing and pulsating from your heart, throughout your body, and into the energy field around your body.
>
> Now feel a shaft of light coming down from above. Call in that light through the crown of your head. Feel the luminous rays fill up your whole body, from the top of your head to the tips of your toes and fingers. Sense the light becoming more incandescent as it then spreads into the energy field around your body. Feel a golden egg of light encompassing and informing you.
>
> Reach your arms and hands out in all directions— above, below, and on both sides—blessing yourself. Then send the blessings to Mother Earth and up to the cosmic canopy, the entire universe.

Afterward, just sit for a moment in the silence and stillness, feeling cleansed and renewed, being love and feeling grateful.

Clean Out Your Gut

Many people with lots of mental body impurities and imbalances experience constipation, diarrhea, or general stomach upset. They also tend to have weight issues, sleep disorders, and self-worth issues. Many studies are suggesting that gut microbes are related to mood, sleep, and weight and that improving your microbiome will help issues in these areas.[3] Each person's situation is unique, but addressing this critical area of gut health is often part of the solution to these problems.

If you've ever considered doing a gut cleanse, days 16 through 20 would be a wonderful time for one, including enemas and colonics. I do "rest and digest" journeys with my rest community because each of the four seasons is a great time to cleanse your system from stagnation that builds up. On a daily basis, you might want to take a good probiotic, drink lots of water, and add fiber-rich foods to your diet.

The Ha Breath

The Ha Breath is one of my favorite breathing practices to help women release strong emotions. The mental body is where you activate the warrior within you, and doing the Ha Breath can help you feel like a warrior. Sometimes I call it the scream-on-a-mountain breath. What woman doesn't want to have a good scream?

I first discovered the Ha Breath while taking a Goddess to the Core workshop with Sierra Bender. What I love about this breath is how it helps you release everything you're holding. It also welcomes masculine energy (step one), feminine energy (step two), and then unites the two (step three), bringing you pretty quickly into a state of oneness. If you begin to feel overwhelmed by any emotions, the Ha Breath is one way to actively release these emotions and come back to a peaceful place.

Here's how to do it.

Step One

1. Begin in a standing position. Lift your hands straight over your head and take a deep breath in through your nose.

2. Squat down and pull your hands into your belly like you're scooping energy from the sky (masculine energy). As you squat, shout out, "Ha!"

3. Return to standing. Repeat three times or more, until you feel complete.

4. Take one minute to feel the vibratory impact on your body and mind.

Step Two

1. Begin in a standing position. Your arms are at your sides. Take a deep breath in through your nose.

2. Squat down and pull your hands up as if you're scooping energy from the earth (feminine energy). As you squat, shout out, "Ha!"

3. Return to standing. Repeat three times or more, until you feel complete.

4. Take one minute to feel the vibratory impact on your body and mind.

Step Three

1. Begin in a standing position. Your arms are at your sides. Take a deep breath in through your nose.

2. Squat down with your hands extended forward, and shout out, "Ha!" as you bring your hands into your belly (uniting masculine and feminine energies).

3. Return to standing. Repeat three times or more, until you feel complete.

4. Take one minute to feel the vibratory impact on your body and mind.

Create a New Intention

These five days are a great time to check in with the intention you're using during yoga nidra meditation. If your intention still feels right, keep it. But if it doesn't, or if your soul whispers have led you to identify an emotion or a recurring situation that you'd like to shift, think of a positive statement for a new intention. This is called a secondary intention. It's more goal oriented but it always relates to your primary intention, which you identified in chapter four. Here are some guidelines developed by John Heister, a senior Amrit Yoga Institute teacher.

Identify a habit or pattern or an area of health, stress, worry, or tension that you'd like to change. To create a new intention around this concern, ask yourself these questions:

What do I want to feel for myself, whether the situation changes or not?

How would I like to be in this situation?

How would it make me feel if I had what I wanted?

Freewrite your answers to these questions. Then look at those answers and notice the key words in them that could be used as a new intention.

For example, Sarah wanted to create an intention that addressed her overeating. For the first question, she wrote that whether she stopped overeating or not, she'd like to "feel more loving" toward herself. In the actual situation, she would like to "be more brave." And then for the final question, she wrote that she would feel "more kind" toward herself. Sarah's new intention became "I am loving, brave, and kind to myself." Notice how her intention didn't mention the actual habit she wanted to release. She knew what habit her intention related to, and that was enough.

Your intention statement does not have to use all the words that resonate with you; instead, make sure it evokes a feeling that resonates. Kiran was having a challenging time parenting her three children. Every day there were intense arguments, particularly with her fourteen-year-old daughter. It was hard for her to even imagine what she wanted to feel for herself, whether the situation changed or not, because she had not thought about her own feelings for a long time. But eventually her answer to question one was "to feel peaceful." For the second question, on how she would want to be in this situation, the words *loving* and *forgiving* stood out. Finally, for the third question, she wrote that if she had what she wanted, a peaceful home with positive communication, she would feel "overjoyed and optimistic." Kiran's new intention became "I am peacefully parenting with love and forgiving myself and my children." She didn't feel the need to include words from her answer to question three because the intention statement itself made her feel optimistic.

Here are some examples of other new intentions women have created in the Release phase:

I am parenting with peaceful language.

I am honest, loving, and forgiving in my relationship.

My body is strong, powerful, and energized.

I feel authentic, confident, and bold at work.

I eat foods that nourish my body and help me feel good.

Remember to phrase your intention as if it were already true, right now. When you establish a new intention, you plant a new seed. What you need to ask yourself now is "What seed do I want to plant to release what's standing in the way of the healthiest version of my self?" A balanced mental body plants only seeds that turn on your internal power switch.

Optional: Diving Deeper

Looking to dive more deeply into warrior energy, darkness, holding opposites, or a new intention? Consider these Daring to Rest optional prompts:

- Freewrite in your journal about your soul whispers.

- Stand in what feels like a warrior position for you—your most confident, courageous self. (It could be one of the warrior poses from yoga or a superhero pose: feet apart, hands on hips, chest forward.) If the warrior in you could speak about her ideal, well-rested life, what would she say? Freewrite about this or record yourself speaking. Then read or listen back to your words.

- Pick a strong emotion you're dealing with in your life now. Freewrite about this emotion and how you feel when you experience it. Then freewrite about the opposite emotion. And finally, freewrite about the two emotions meeting. You can also express these emotions and their meeting through movement or in a drawing.

- Sit in the dark, indoors or outdoors, for five minutes. Then freewrite about darkness. Say as much as you can about how darkness made you feel and anything else on what darkness means to you.

- If your new intention were a song, what song would it be? Your song could be real or an imagined title. Dance to your song, imagining your intention taking place.

Key Points in Chapter Seven

- Your mental body is the third of five bodies of awareness that reside in you. It does the deep cleaning of your mind.

- A balanced mental body helps you go from disconnected and numb to powerful.

- One of the most powerful yoga nidra practices is Holding Opposites. It can help you transform out of negative habits and patterns and begin to water the seed of new habits and patterns that help you turn on your internal power switch.

8

WISDOM

Becoming the Witness of Your Life

Days 21–25

What if you could take a step back and begin to see your life as if you're watching it, not in it? This is exactly what begins to happen in the wisdom body, the fourth body of awareness accessed in yoga nidra. After clearing blocks in your mental body, your mind begins to see more clearly, ego moves aside, and you begin to access your inner knowing.

For the next five days, the goal is to tap into your intuition and awareness beyond your everyday life. The wisdom body is where the wise woman in you whispers, *You've got this.* Writing, painting, and doing math are activities that can connect us to the wisdom body. While the mental body balances your ordinary mind, the wisdom body balances your higher mind, the place where you see your real self and download new insights. When life gets difficult, a balanced wisdom body helps you take a step back and become the peaceful observer of your life. You feel everything in your life, but you no longer become undone by challenges.

Basic Instructions for Days 21 to 25

1. Practice the Phase Two: Release Meditation daily. Continue to use your most recent intention statement and hold your touchstone in your left hand when practicing, or if it feels right, place your touchstone on the space between your eyebrows or any place that needs healing.

2. Continue to listen for and track your soul whispers.

3. Practice connecting with your Council of Women and feeling their guidance, using the instructions in this chapter.

4. Optional: Use additional practices to connect with and balance your wisdom body.

5. Optional: Use the prompts to get to know your Wild Woman, explore your intuition, and dive more deeply into other concepts from this chapter.

The Power of the Wisdom Body

The wisdom body is the place of symbols, colors, visions, and dreams. During your yoga nidra meditation, when you're introduced to images and symbols or visualization, you are balancing the wisdom body. You may notice in the Phase Two: Release Meditation that you are guided to a bonfire on a beach; in the Phase Three: Rise Meditation, you will be guided to a temple. Why? Because it's in the wisdom body that you can take a step back from your ego, thoughts begin to recede, and all the ways you look at your thoughts as right or wrong and all the ways you see yourself as separate from others begin to fade. In the wisdom body, the mind stops lecturing you, and you drop into a soothing place in the nervous system.

Visualization and holding opposites guides you to a place where you stop believing that your thoughts make things happen, and instead the wanting to make things happen comes out of the mystery of life. You're in wonder. When yoga nidra uses visualization, it often guides you to places in nature because in nature it's easier to wonder, to let go of our thoughts.

Then, when you wake from yoga nidra and continue with your daily life, this awareness allows you to stop taking everything so personally. You still have plenty of thoughts in your everyday life because thoughts do serve you, enabling you to do things like eat and pay taxes. But because of your yoga nidra experience, you also now begin to view life with detached awareness, like it's a movie, and this reduces how much everyday life controls and drains you. You stop engaging in draining interactions because you stop expecting anyone, including yourself, to fix your personal story. You're no longer the victim of your story. Instead, you can now hear any healing messages. In a yoga nidra visualization, you will often be invited to feel sensations in your body and to see if there is a healing or creative message for you. You can begin to heal when you hear this message. You begin to become the heroine of your story.

The wisdom body is a deep level of consciousness that is not easy to access in everyday life. During your yoga nidra meditation, it takes a minimum of ten minutes to enter this state. It's the place from which composers and writers create great works of art. The more the first three bodies are in balance, the easier it is to access this peaceful space. While I'm sure there are some people who experience a balanced wisdom body naturally, few can maintain this awareness every day. Mostly, wisdom body awareness comes in waves, increasing the more you meditate or engage in other things that give rise to wonder. Then one day you find you're not so bothered by your external world. The dramas can happen, but you don't feel so intensely about them because you've created a solid foundation that is rooted in intuition, the mental body, and higher-mind consciousness, the wisdom body. It's here that the deeper levels of emotional exhaustion drop. Is life perfect? No. You will feel sad and angry and tired some days. But a purified wisdom body will allow you to meet and feel your thoughts and go beyond them. This is deeply freeing because you're essentially free to awaken to your most pure, authentic self. You get out of your own way. The most effective leaders, and well-rested ones, have "awakened" moments, when ego and all the thoughts that go with it are not there.

Women practicing yoga nidra have different experiences while clearing their wisdom bodies, but typically as the wisdom body balances, they feel a deep sense of peace. Deborah, whom you met in the introduction to "Phase Two: Release," bravely traveled an imperfect path that felt like a relentless struggle to find peace as she grieved the loss of her life partner. She practiced yoga nidra meditation daily—and sometimes twice per day—for months, until finally she began to take a tiny step back from her grief, rather than let it consume her everyday life.

As the wisdom body begins to balance, we tend to receive soul whispers with powerful, life-changing messages, or images with such messages may come outside of our yoga nidra practice. After five months, Deborah one day received an image at the end of her yoga nidra practice. She saw herself and her beloved with a Native American blanket wrapped around them on the beach. It was like a memory—very physical. She could hear the ocean and his heartbeat. The next day after yoga nidra meditation, she had another vision: both she and her beloved were again on the beach, but this time he was invisible. When she leaned back, it was like he was a ghost. Deborah felt lots of sadness, but she could also feel things shifting. Then in her vision, she realized she had joined with him, like they were one.

On day three, after yoga nidra meditation, she saw herself looking out at the ocean. "There I was," she told me, "I was a wise woman—and my beloved was gone." Deborah felt relief that he was okay. And for the first time in many months, she didn't feel scared to be alone, which had been a big theme for her after he had died. Instead, in her vision, she was carrying the Native American blanket, and she felt like she was a carrier of something really precious.

"It's then that I realized I'm carrying the legacy of our love forward," she shared. This was deeply powerful for her. As she notes, "The question when you lose a loved one is always, 'Where are they?' In this vision, I had reinforcement that my beloved is everywhere. He is the rain; he is on the sand."

The visions Deborah received after yoga nidra for those three days were a progression from "he's here" to "he's everywhere." She knows he is okay, but the truth is, she doesn't know where he is. Instead, she now knows the place where she holds him. This is the life-changing magic that can come when your wisdom body begins to balance. Ego, finally, begins to fall away.

The End of Ego and Rise of the True Self

Ego is the voice within that says "I," "me," and "mine." It is the voice that tells us we are separate from others. We need ego to survive, but separation is what we must transcend to feel peaceful and whole. The ultimate goal of a spiritual path is to open the door to the oneness of all. When you are lying down practicing yoga nidra meditation, this is the tune-up you're getting. You're being guided to a timeless state of being where ego falls away. You could see this in Deborah's story. For many months, she felt separate from others. This was ego at work. But the moment her wisdom body began to come into balance, she began to feel whole again.

The slippery slope with ego is that it causes you to beat up on yourself: *I'm not pretty. I'm not enough. I'm not worthy.* If you're grieving and you feel you're not doing it right, that's ego. When a friend gets a great job and you hate your job and you're jealous, that's ego. Comparing yourself to others is a destructive form of ego. I can sometimes get myself in this loop, and so does every other woman who comes into my yoga nidra programs. We all say, "It feels icky." This is because when we feel separate, we have a feeling of isolation. Many spiritual traditions, especially Buddhism, say ego is an illusion, a false way we identify ourselves. It's really hard to comprehend this when we're in the comparison loop or when we have had a bad experience, like getting up in front of a crowd and doing a bad job and then living in that criticism of ourselves and never going on a stage again. Ego can and does stop us from being brave. I see it all the time.

Compare this ego loop to how you feel after you practice yoga nidra meditation. Most women tell me they feel "completely open," "honest," "all love," and "dreamy." This is ego falling away. Every time you lie down to practice yoga nidra and are guided to the wisdom body, your mind is trained to become a witness. It also helps to melt—at least temporarily, when you first practice—the feeling of separateness from others. This is the beginning of freedom from the isolation and fear that ego fosters.

Once ego loosens its grip, our true, authentic self rises. We're then able to use our wisdom to determine when ego is serving us and when it's not serving us. Training your mind to become the witness of your life allows you to be objective about what the mind and ego tell you. Many of the reasons you thought "I can't" fall away, and you begin to feel limitless.

I love this moment when a woman feels she can do anything. For years, Margreet, whom you read about in chapters four and five, was stuck in a mental loop of anger over her childhood, particularly her relationship with her mother. The moment she dropped her anger, and the thoughts associated with it, she could take a step back and become the witness of her life. This loosened ego's hold, which propelled her to express exactly who she was—her real self. She had practiced yoga nidra meditation for seven months, and then one day, she emailed me to say, "I am taking steps to start my own business, to live my passion, to go out there and help everybody—with my energy." She was taking these steps after receiving a clear message during her yoga nidra meditation to start her own business. "And yoga nidra is such a big part of the trust I feel to take these steps," she said.

I commonly see women who have been playing small gain the courage to play big the moment they become the witness. It's a beautiful transformation and not an unusual one to experience when you are practicing yoga nidra meditation. The limitless feeling that results from becoming the witness releases many women from the fear of playing big. I also see these women using this limitless feeling as fuel to be successful on a new set of terms—one that honors all of themselves, not just their ego-driven desires. For example, a woman who was pushed into being a lawyer might decide to open an art gallery because that's what sings to her true self. A consistent yoga nidra practice makes it almost impossible to not open to life's options in ways you never imagined.

Let me be clear: ego isn't bad. A healthy ego doesn't bound itself in your personality or in thoughts and emotions. Instead, it knows that the "me" who you are when you are called by your name is a small fraction of the "me" living inside you. It doesn't get attached to your daily wins and losses. Your healthy ego knows that it lives and functions in your body, but it's free from the need to become anything. A consistently balanced wisdom body gives us access to this healthy ego, so it's possible to sense a deeper presence in the body and mind, a connection to the universal law that all is one. The moment you sense this, another layer of exhaustion lifts, and a familiar part of you, a part you had turned your back on, shows up.

Here Comes Your Wild Woman

Who is this familiar part of you? She is robust, brave, and intuitive. You often sense her while spending time in nature. When you connect back to her, you feel something stirring in you, like you've touched the essence of who you are. This is your Wild Woman.

I began to notice that women, after practicing yoga nidra meditation for a few weeks, often said it felt "like I've stepped into a new world that's more real to me—a deeper truth of who I am," and "like I'm strengthening muscle memory of who I really am." They often told me that they now take time each month during their menstruation to cry or journal. Older women often said they feel unafraid to be honest with people or to finally finish the novel they have mapped out in their mind. I'd hear in a pregnant woman's voice a confidence about giving birth that wasn't initially there. The Wild Woman had arisen in each of these women.

Dr. Clarissa Pinkola Estés made the Wild Woman archetype well known through her book *Women Who Run With the Wolves*. According to Pinkola Estés, the Wild Woman often rises when you begin to tune in to your intuition and tell your stories truthfully. The Wild Woman is completely in touch with her natural rhythms and cycles. She is unafraid to show her healer and spiritual self. She usually comes forth when a woman can access a higher level of consciousness, which is exactly what happens when your wisdom body is consistently balanced.

When you first lay down to practice yoga nidra meditation, especially if you felt like the worn-out woman, you were most likely disconnected from your Wild Woman. Our busy world, both the pace and the lack of connection to nature, can cause our intuition, our wise self, to go into hiding. We begin to question our decisions. We let ourselves be preyed on because we aren't in touch with our Wild Woman instinct, which would tell us an absolute no or yes. In yoga nidra, balancing the first and second bodies of awareness—the physical body and energy body—begins to wake up your Wild Woman, and listening for your soul whispers does too. But to truly reunite with your Wild Woman, you need to continue going inward.

In the mental body, you meet and greet the dark sides of you, so you can then see the light. Once you begin to see the light, your internal world opens, you have access to the wisdom body, where ego falls away and your Wild Woman is given permission to flourish because the Wild Woman sees a world without separation. She doesn't need anything to change. She knows that the ground underneath us never goes away, so there is no need to be afraid of falling; you can close your eyes and feel safe.

Most women meet some version of their Wild Woman in the wisdom body. I like to imagine it like this: while you are in the wisdom body, your Wild Woman takes your worn-out woman clothes away from you, and she hands you a clean, well-rested woman outfit. Then, as Pinkola Estés puts it, you begin to listen to everything in life with "soul-hearing."[1]

Your Wild Woman is the original rebel, the original revolutionary. She is feared by patriarchy and any establishment doctrine because she simply won't put up with being put down. Worn-out women wear that legacy like a badge, but the Wild Woman simply won't. She is connected to her deep inner knowing. The reason she surfaces now is because in the wisdom body you finally understand the duality of life: that life is not about *either-or*—either I'm happy or I'm sad. Rather, it is often *both-and*—that you can be both happy and sad. Your Wild Woman gets this because she is the personification of duality. She has an outer life that's practical, and she also has an inner life that is about feeling and deeper knowing.

To the outside world, this duality can seem confusing and irritating, and women get judged for being too emotional or sensitive. But when you touch your wisdom body more and more, you begin to see that this sensitive side has an opposite, so referring to you as "too sensitive" doesn't tell the whole story. As Pinkola Estés explains, this "twin nature" of women, this "two-women-who-are-one," may baffle others.[2] It might baffle us as well, but much of our struggle as women has been to understand this wildish nature ourselves, to not push it away, and to have others understand it. We rebel precisely because we feel our essential nature is misunderstood, and constantly struggling with this misunderstanding is exhausting.

Even when you're exhausted, your Wild Woman is there. The problem is that the moment she is taken out of the role of heroine, through physical or psychological oppression—as she was during the industrial revolution, when women were told that they should be happy wives only, or today, when women see they are not being paid equally for their work—she begins to die. While women have a history of being used for men's enjoyment—as his counsel, to mother him, or make his life easier—actually, in our ancient memories, mostly before the ancient Egyptians ruled, women were celebrated for their power, seen as true matriarchs. Our more recent history has led women to hide their Wild Woman, our highly intuitive selves, and as a result, we are exhausted. Why? Because women who lead—at home and work—in ways that do not elevate their Wild Woman are disconnected from their internal power switches. They can be successful, but at a cost, and the cost is often ignoring their Wild Woman, who is, ironically, their means of not just leading, but also of thriving.

If you're not going into deep sleep often, your Wild Woman is not being fed, and you may continue to feel exhausted. I am convinced that this is why so many women have a very powerful, almost teary-eyed reaction when they discover yoga nidra meditation. It not only gives them permission to sleep deeply again and lie down, but it also puts them back in touch with their Wild Woman.

Connect to Your Council of Women

The great news is that during yoga nidra, what I call your Council of Women will often appear to help you stay connected to your Wild Woman. Your personal Council of Women is typically made up of female messengers or guides who come to you in a spiritual, not physical, form. Think of them as mentors. While you don't consciously choose them, they often appear when you call for them toward the end of yoga nidra. They might be strong women you've known, like grandmothers or other female relations who have passed on. They may also be women you don't know personally, such as powerful women you admire from history. They might even include the living women you respect. One woman in my rest program, for example, had a Council of Women that included her mother who had passed away, her two closest girlfriends, a business mentor, and well-known actress Meryl Streep. Another woman had no one familiar, but the women who came all arrived wearing the same blue color, her favorite color as a child. Often your Council of Women, like yoga nidra, helps point you toward freedom.

Consulting your Council of Women is a way to consult the wise woman in you, reconnect to your inner knowing, and receive guidance. This practice is sometimes hard for women to grasp because you have to believe in what you can't see. But once you get the hang of it, calling on your Council of Women is actually quick, easy, and deeply meaningful. If you're like most women, you'll love this practice because, finally, it feels as though a group of wise women have your back.

As you already know, the Phase Two: Release Meditation specifically asks you to call in your Council of Women, so you may already feel familiar with them. From now through the final day of the Daring to Rest program, I suggest that you also practice calling in your Council of Women *outside of* the yoga nidra meditations. This is a quick and easy way to stay in touch with your inner world. You don't have do this practice every day, but please do it as often as possible.

Here's how: Close your eyes, put your right and left hands over your heart, and ask your Council of Women to assemble. You can also imagine sending out a signal, such as a color or sound, and then watch them appear. Or first practice the Open Your Feminine Highway technique in chapter five. They may appear as images in your mind, or you'll just receive an internal knowing that your Council of Women has arrived. This takes only a few minutes. The trick is to stay silent, breathe slowly, and imagine them assembling.

Once your Council of Women has assembled, feel how they accept and bless exactly who you are. You don't need to do anything else other than receive this blessing from them, but if you're in a healing crisis or difficult situation, you may wish to ask them a question. It could be a direct question, such as, "How can I have less pain during menstruation?" or a more open question, like, "How can I feel more peaceful?" Ask them about an area of your life where you feel stressed. Don't tell them a story; they already know all your stories. Just ask and wait for the answer. They may have questions in return. You can answer them, but try to be more in deep-listening mode after you ask your question. Let your Council of Women provide guidance.

My Council of Women is usually three women, and when I close my eyes, they appear in my mind's eye, sitting on couches, looking very relaxed. The actual women who show up have changed over the years, so don't be expecting your Council of Women to always consist of the same women every time you call on them. Some women I know have many more than three show up; others have fewer. Expect your experience to be unique to you.

If you're not convinced you need a Council of Women or think it's too "woo-woo," let me share why you might want to reconsider. Deep down, you always know what action to take in your life, and know who you are, but sometimes you need a force within you to reveal it to you. This force is your Council of Women. They are the awakened part of you. When you practice yoga nidra, you're resting into the awareness of who you are, and this opens you to seeing who you are not. Your Council of Women gives you the extra support you need to see clearly. They're the transition team between yoga nidra (your inner world), and your everyday life (your outer world). They help you figure out what to give attention to in your life and what to withdraw attention from.

The great news is that when you've been practicing yoga nidra meditation regularly and calling on your Council of Women, they will make themselves available quite readily in your everyday life.

Another way of connecting to your Council of Women is with guidance cards. You can buy decks of guidance cards that depict feminine archetypes or goddesses. These feminine archetypes reveal human traits, meanings, values, and motives that exist within most women's psyches. When we see these archetypes, they often help us tap into our Wild Woman nature. They can also help us understand our behaviors and patterns.

If you'd prefer to make your own deck of guidance cards, use your soul whispers. Simply write your soul whispers from days 1 through 20 on separate pieces of paper or index cards.

If one day you aren't able to practice yoga nidra or call in your Council of Women, you can simply pick a guidance card instead. First, hold all the cards (or soul whisper papers) in your hands and ask that they be used for your highest good and the highest good of humanity. Then spread out the cards. Take a slow, deep breath and pick a card with your left hand. Read the meaning of the card you receive and notice how it relates to your life. Sense what the card is asking of you.

Picking a daily guidance card is great for women who are having women's health issues—anything from menstrual problems to fertility issues—because even though these are the moments when it's important to slow down and connect to our Wild Woman, we usually feel overwhelmed with solving our health issue and can fall out of sync with her at these times. This is exactly when you need your Council of Women. Using your guidance cards to reconnect to your inner knowing can take a lot of pressure off you during a very tense period.

Optional: Additional Practices for Your Wisdom Body

During days 21 through 25, it's important to not engage in activities that are particularly competitive because this can feed your ego and take you away from connection to your true self. This includes athletic yoga asana practices. The practices and activities that follow are some ways you can balance the wisdom body both during and outside of your yoga nidra practice.

Activate Your Soul

The wisdom body is connected to your soul, not to a specific power center. To increase intuition and feel a connection with your Wild Woman, you may wish to place your touchstone on the space between your eyebrows (your third eye) during your yoga nidra meditation or on an area of your body that you feel needs healing or creative energy. You might also like to use a few drops of citrus or cypress essential oils on your clothes or inhale it from your hands. Wearing white or indigo helps activate the soul.

So Hum Breath

This is a beloved breathing meditation that many women find deeply relaxing because it connects you back to a higher state of consciousness and gives you access to your true self. *So Hum* is a Sanskrit phrase that means "I am that." This phrase plugs you back into "all that is" in the universe. You can sit or lie down to practice this meditation. An ideal practice time is ten or more minutes, but just a few rounds will make a difference. Here's how to do it:

1. Take five deep, slow breaths through the nose. Imagine the breath going in and out of the space between your eyebrows—your third eye. This will oxygenate your blood and relax your body.

2. Now, from your third eye, inhale slowly, imagining the breath traveling down to the base of your spine. At the same time, mentally say the sound *Soooooo*.

3. Slowly exhale while imagining the breath moving from the base of the spine back up to the third eye. At the same time, silently saying the sound *Hummmmmm*.

4. Feel your awareness expanding and merging with divine energy.

5. Continue to silently chant *Soooooo Hummmmmm* in rhythm with your inhales and exhales.

6. At the end, focus your attention on your third eye for a moment and feel the vibration of sensation in your body.

Tapping Your Thymus

Tapping your thymus is a simple practice you can do just before going to sleep or any time during the day to bring yourself to a more peaceful, open place. The thymus gland is located in the center of the chest, beneath the breastbone (sternum). If you feel nervous or stressed, tapping this place lightly with the knuckles a few times will bring you back into balance again. Tapping the thymus is particularly useful when you are going through a difficult time. It reminds you to shake ego's hold on your emotions and thoughts.

Optional: Diving Deeper

Looking to dive more deeply into your Wild Woman? Consider these Daring to Rest optional prompts:

- Describe your Wild Woman. If your Wild Woman were a color, what color would she be? If she had a name, what would her name be? Freewrite about her.

- Express your Wild Woman through movement while listening to a song of your choice.

- Draw or paint your Wild Woman. Show lots of detail, similar to an anatomical drawing.

- If your Wild Woman could speak, what would she say? Freewrite as if you are your Wild Woman speaking.

- Freewrite in your journal about your soul whispers.

Key Points in Chapter Eight

- Your wisdom body is the fourth of the five bodies of awareness that reside in you. It is the seat of your inner knowing and higher mind.

- During yoga nidra meditation, you are guided through the wisdom body to access a timeless space where the grip of ego falls away. This provides peace of mind and access to your intuition.

- As you balance your wisdom body, a familiar, robust Wild Woman emerges. The more you embrace her, the more you begin to shed the worn-out woman.

9

BLISS

Knowing Everything Is Okay

Days 26-30

The moment I love the most during yoga nidra meditation is toward the end, when you're barely sensing your body, all thoughts fade, your heart opens, and this sense of being connected to a universal fire emerges. Whether there's something going on in your personal life or at work or in the world, you feel all boundaries dissolve, and an unshakeable sense that "all is right with the world" infuses every cell and atom, like an intravenous drip of love and compassion. You feel a powerful connection with humanity, a peaceful knowing of your infinite depth. You're deeply asleep, often with zero thoughts—in your unconscious mind, in some sense virtually dead—and at the same time wildly alive, as if you're in the transition stage of giving birth. There is a total absence of pleasure and pain in your mind. This is the fifth and final body of awareness: the bliss body.

Basic Instructions for Days 26 to 30

1. Practice the Phase Two: Release Meditation daily.
   Continue to use your most recent intention statement.
   Also continue to hold your touchstone in your left
   hand when practicing, or you may wish to place your
   touchstone on your heart.

2. Continue to listen for and track your soul whispers.

3. Optional: Continue to practice connecting with your
   Council of Women both during yoga nidra and outside
   of your yoga nidra meditation.

4. Optional: Use the additional practices in this chapter
   to balance your bliss body.

5. Optional: Use the Diving Deeper prompts to explore
   concepts in this chapter, including bliss, who you truly
   are, and sharing a difficult story.

Following Your Bliss Body

One of my favorite thinkers is mythologist and writer Joseph Campbell, whose work is often summarized by his phrase, "Follow your bliss." Great quote, but when most people think of the meaning of *bliss*, they think it means they should book that trip to Bali. Nope. Bliss is about more than just pleasure. In the bliss body, you notice that your awareness can expand way beyond you, to infinity, and it's this awareness that tears your heart wide open. This is a huge moment for many people during the practice of yoga nidra because it's when the small self in you steps aside and the big self shows up. You feel a sense of freedom and expansiveness. You start showing up with love and compassion more easily in all situations in your life. In the bliss body, you can access all of the qualities of the heart—bliss, peace, harmony, love, understanding, empathy, clarity, unity, compassion, kindness, and forgiveness.

It is rumored that later in his career, as a lecturer at Sarah Lawrence College, Campbell was so dismayed by the misinterpretation of the word *bliss* that he said he should have told people to "follow their blisters." The good news is that's exactly what you've been doing in yoga nidra meditation—meeting and greeting emotional "blisters"—which is why you're now well primed to balance the bliss body.

I nearly did a yoga nidra backflip when I read that Campbell's concept of bliss came from the same spiritual teachings as yoga nidra meditation. Campbell noticed that in Sanskrit there is a well-known term, *satchitananda*, which means "the essence of the divine self that lives within you." This word breaks down to three words: *sat, chit,* and *ananda. Sat* means "truth," *chit* means "consciousness," and *ananda* means "bliss." Campbell believed the easiest concept for people to understand was ananda, and he told people to "follow your bliss" because if we did, truth and consciousness would follow. Unfortunately, many people didn't get it; they didn't see that bliss is an inside job.

To access bliss, instead of flying to Bali, the journey you must make is to your inner world. If you don't, then bliss is seen through the eyes of ego, and you begin grabbing at material things—like a hammock with the perfect ocean view in Bali—and expect they will bring long-term pleasure. In yoga nidra, every time you practice, you travel to your inner world, and it's here that truth and consciousness are activated via the wisdom body. You start to see the truth of who you are and what the world around you is—no more illusions—and this then gives rise to bliss.

The bliss body feeds your big self, not your small self. Women tell me that during the bliss body part of a yoga nidra meditation, they feel this floating-on-air feeling or that their heart opens beyond the boundaries of their body. One woman told me that she felt it "allowed me to see who I am no matter where I am in work or where I live." One woman told me that she felt "reconnected to my essence," and another said she felt "the deepest peace in my body and outside my body." Such feelings and sensations are your bliss body being scrubbed clean, the final layer of emotional exhaustion letting go. In this moment, you turn on your internal power switch, making yourself fully available for health and wholeness.

A balanced bliss body allows you to recognize that the source of love is within you. This understanding comes because you are in the deepest state of sleep, below the ego and mind, in the unconscious. This place is like a Garden of Eden, where unity and oneness flourish. Your body is relaxed and at total peace. And it's here you viscerally learn the secrets of achieving deep peace in your everyday life. Sleep problems, as well as health issues, are resolved here because you're connected to the source within you. You're an ocean, not a wave anymore, and this understanding connects you to a higher power, turning darkness into light. You're no longer afraid of your light. Now you are who you are, which is when the final veil of exhaustion lifts. You realize how tired you were from looking for yourself everywhere, and finally you are free. You have calmed your outer senses, and now the inner flame is lit—a deep love within—and you're connected to a universal fire, to all humans and nonhumans. As you cleanse the bliss body, all of this is downloaded into your being.

The bliss body is your deepest, most subtle layer of being—your core existence, a consciousness that's beyond the limits of the body. It's here you begin to feel into a state of being that has always existed but was buried by the other four bodies. Accessing the bliss body removes the final thin layer of illusion, and once it is lifted, you are able to see the pureness of your soul.

This timeless state of being does occasionally appear to us in our outer world, such as when we're holding a newborn baby, watching a birth, painting, or writing a poem. All of these things touch the bliss body. These experiences make us feel alive, full of possibility, open, spacious, and feathery light. Who can look at a healthy newborn baby and not feel their heart open and a hope for the future? Everything feels like it's okay. Most likely, you've had at least a few these experiences during your life.

I tell women who have a hard time with the concepts of bliss and joy to start with noticing in their bodies and minds this sense that "it's going to be okay." What if you could give yourself permission to start here? If you've experienced trauma or any form of abuse, or you've been worn out for a long time, it may feel like a huge leap to sense that all is okay with the world. Many times you can't go to that kind of bliss right away, but you can slowly feel into this sense that everything is okay. While not everyone with trauma will have a hard time sensing bliss, some people have a freeze response that helps them deal with the moment of trauma, and after the trauma they stay in a disassociated-reaction mode as a means of coping. Remember to lovingly meet yourself wherever you are. Once the sense that everything is going to be okay feels normal, you'll often be able to go a little deeper to gratitude for everything, and then you'll slowly begin to feel bliss.

A Fourth State of Sleep

As you practice yoga nidra meditation, eventually, in the bliss body, you enter a deep meditative state like a spiritual trance. This is a fourth state of sleep known as *turiya*. According to the Upanishads (among the oldest of India's spiritual texts), there are four fundamental states that every person has access to: waking, dreaming, deep sleep, and turiya. We can experience the first three through our normal waking and sleeping. We function in our waking world in the conscious mind; in the dream world, we function in the subconscious mind; and during deep sleep, we enter the unconscious mind. Turiya is a fourth state of sleep, in which you can access supreme stillness and deep healing. It is said that turiya is the seer, and the three other states are illusions because they appear and disappear. So to know your true self at its core, you must access turiya. This fourth state can be realized through yoga nidra and other forms of deep meditation, but it's impossible to enter it through conventional sleep.

People who consistently experience turiya are able to tap into their potential of genius because they have access to a deep state of awakening. In turiya, your thoughts stop. Your unconscious mind is completely at rest and fertile, able to absorb affirmations and intentions without judgment or fear.

You may have noticed that many athletes go into an altered state while doing their sport, so they are able to operate with deep clarity, overcome adversity, and focus on their goals. They forget about time or being hungry or injured, and instead operate in a zone of inspiration. Writers enter this zone and create masterpieces from here. It is often said that Gandhi, who meditated and prayed every morning at 4:30 am, was liberated by turiya. In his autobiography, he described being in a meditative state throughout his day and how even in difficult times he felt inspired. People had great faith in Gandhi primarily because they knew he was operating from an absolute awakened level.

I think of turiya as not only a delicious fourth state of consciousness and deep stillness that you can experience in your yoga nidra meditation, but also a dimension of universal love. One woman told me that she felt so at peace after practicing yoga nidra that it was as if she were "becoming one with God." This is when I knew she had touched turiya. In our busy lives, we forget that divine energy is always there for us, and when we do, we suffer. We feel exhausted, and we experience pain. Disconnection from the divine is the ultimate form of exhaustion.

Whether I say *God* or *divine energy*, neither is about believing in a religion. The divine is the essence of everything. In yoga nidra, after purifying all five bodies, you are now connected with the most intimate, vulnerable, tender, gentle part of the soul of a human being, unshielded by the defenses of the other four bodies. Your internal power switch is on. You are one with the divine. The reason many of us engage in religious practices, like prayer and chanting, is that they help us go inward and feel a oneness with the divine. It's in this moment, face-to-face with your soul, the closest you can come to the essence of everything, that you know undeniably that everything will be okay.

God Is Waiting for You
(Everything Is Going to Be Okay)

I don't speak about the divine or God easily. I wasn't brought up with much religion, but there's something about life falling apart that leads us back to the divine. If you have experienced or are experiencing post-traumatic stress disorder (PTSD), or a challenging moment in your life, you understand how hard it is to have faith when you don't feel peaceful inside and how hard it is to connect back to a universal channel of love.

I want to tell you a story about my life that is not easy to tell. When bad things happen, there's this wave of emotions we feel, and that wave can keep crashing over us even years later when the story of what happened to us threatens to be replayed or retold. Sometimes just thinking about the story can overwhelm our system. The beauty of yoga nidra is that when you experience oneness with the divine again and again, one day you wake up feeling braver than ever before, ready to tell the hard story and ready to release a deep layer of the pain and suffering.

In 2007, my husband and I decided we were going to live our dream life: to return to Africa to live with our children. My husband lived in parts of Africa as a child, and we had lived in Kenya together before we had children. Now I was nearly forty, we had two kids, and we wanted to head back. We made vision boards of our dream location, a little town in Tanzania that had a nice international school and is situated right on the gateway to the Serengeti game park. West of this town is the Ngorongoro Crater, the world's largest inactive, intact, and unfilled volcanic crater, full of wildlife—lions, wildebeests, zebras—and named "Gift of Life" by the local Masai people. Our vision board had all of this on it. We dreamed of raising our children here. My husband, who works in international development, received several job leads in other places in Africa, but since our older son had dyslexia, we had to be picky and only go to a place where he could get services. So we held out. And one day, not too long after we created our vision board, out of the blue, my husband was offered a job in the town we had envisioned living. Three months later, we sold everything, said good-bye to family and friends, and left to follow our dream.

Our dream actually included another vision: we would live in Tanzania with Faith, a Kenyan friend. Have you ever had that moment when you meet someone and you know they are one of the people you will hold dear forever? This was my experience with Faith. She had been our maid when we'd lived in Kenya, but really, other than income separation and a life lived on different continents and communities, she was one of my people. She used to sweep her way toward me in our apartment in Nairobi to tell me that she was never going to marry a Kenyan man because they treat women like doormats—and she was no doormat. One day she told me that she believes men are like heads and women are like necks. "Everyone thinks the head controls everything," she'd say, "but really the neck controls the head."

I loved Faith's version of feminism, and I loved her character. She clearly knew who she was: a strong Christian woman, with a great sense of humor, who had deep faith and unfaltering hope. When we moved to Tanzania, the bonus dream was for Faith to join us. She would live in our home again—this time as family. And so it was. She took a five-hour bus from Kenya to our home in Tanzania, she met my boys for the first time, and we were reunited. Life couldn't have been better. I was in a great place professionally. I had a very successful play that had just premiered in multiple locations around the world. We were happy.

Then, one night after my husband had driven a friend to the airport and arrived back at our house late at night, everything changed. We were robbed. Violently. Three armed African men with guns escorted my husband into our house. First they took our wedding rings—mine a simple gold ring given to me by my husband's mother before she died, a ring that had traveled to the women in his family for generations. Next they took me upstairs and asked me to give them all of our money. Then they asked for any guns we had in the house, but we didn't have any. After that, they requested all my jewelry. I gave them everything I could find, remembering their words as they passed the bedroom where my kids were sleeping: "If you do anything stupid, we'll kill you and your motherfucking children." Luckily, when they wanted to force me into the trunk of our car, now their getaway vehicle, my husband convinced them this would not work. They eventually brought me back inside the house and left me tied up on the floor. We were all tied up with telephone and computer cords on the floor—my husband, me, the night watchman, and Faith.

Before the robbers left, they got Faith up from the floor and took her first into the kitchen, then into her bedroom, and finally back to the floor. Once they left, just after midnight, we managed to free ourselves. The first words Faith said to me were, "God is good, Karen. They did not harm the children." Then we held each other in an embrace for a long time. Her next words were, "I need to see a doctor." Faith had been raped. I couldn't believe it. How she could hold hope (because the kids were fine) and hopelessness (having been raped) at the same time? But that was Faith, always holding opposites. I remember her whispering to me, "Everything is going to be okay, Karen. We are alive. The kids are alive. Thank God."

I didn't understand this at the time, how Faith had chosen light over darkness, but I do now. My light was getting dimmer, especially after we woke the children and, under the dark night sky, escorted by dozens of security guards holding AK-47s, we left our home and traveled to a hotel, not knowing our future. The boys were told we had been robbed, but they were also told we were all asleep when it happened. Nobody was hurt. We were okay. I repeated Faith's words to them, "Everything's going to be okay," in the way a mother is supposed to do to reassure them that they were safe, but the truth was, I didn't feel everything was going to be okay. I didn't feel at all.

The next day, we made our way to the police precinct, and then I took Faith to a medical clinic to have a physical exam and start pills for preventing AIDS and pregnancy. It was the worst day of my life. And yet Faith wore a shirt that read, "Jesus Loves Me." I know now that this was her freedom cry. What was mine? I had none. I only saw darkness. I remember seeing Faith's shirt and feeling envious and angry. Outwardly, I thought it was ridiculous to mention Jesus loving you the day after you'd been raped. Inwardly, in the part of me that still had hope, I wished she had another shirt for me.

We had been robbed on Thursday, and on Sunday Faith asked us to take her to a church. I thought of practicing yoga nidra while she was at church, but instead, I sat on the hotel bed eating a plate of french fries. I wasn't ready to feel. In the coming weeks, I stopped practicing yoga nidra, and after a few months, and then years, I had forgotten all about yoga nidra.

How could I forget it, my favorite rest tool for years? I forgot because I got caught in the too-busy cycle. We lived in a hotel for a month with small children, ages five and seven. They started school. I thought Faith needed me more than I needed me. So I pushed yoga nidra away for a long time. And slowly I sank into total darkness. I had post-traumatic stress for two years following Tanzania. We returned to the United States with no possessions because we had sold everything to realize our dream of living in Africa. The stock market crashed. Jobs were scarce. We had no home, little money, and no income. Our dream was over.

Also, we had left Faith in Africa. I'd felt my heart breaking when we left her. How could we leave her? How could we stay? No choice seemed right. All roads seemed to lead to darkness.

For two years after Tanzania, I remained in darkness. I was afraid of random people, the night. I saw the robbers' Doc Martens boots in my sleep every night. Until one day, I remembered what I had forgotten: yoga nidra meditation. I was not trained in it yet, but I had been practicing it before Tanzania, and it had made a huge difference in my life. I began to lie down again with my old friend yoga nidra, setting the simple intention, "I feel." Day by day, month by month, I found my way back to the light.

That's when I knew: everything *is* going to be okay. In Faith's words, "Jesus loves me." I now see that being able to remember "Jesus loves me" is the moment in yoga nidra, in the bliss body, when the spark of your life force and the flame of your soul come closest. Out of this moment comes bliss, a time to integrate what we experience. Some call this grace. When you practice yoga nidra regularly after a difficult time or trauma, this is what happens. You integrate what you experience instead of letting it consume you. You feel all the darkness, and you also feel the light. You open to grace. Yoga nidra leads you back to your internal power switch, where there is no longer an either-or option. You begin to live in the both-and mode. Yes, I was robbed, and I am now safe. The moment I felt this viscerally through yoga nidra, the post-traumatic stress and night fears went away. Gone. Vanished.

After Tanzania, I became trained in iRest yoga nidra meditation and certified in the Amrit Method of yoga nidra. During the Amrit training, our instructor, Yogi Amrit Desai, gave a beautiful talk about yoga nidra, and at the end he said that yoga nidra gives you God's email and phone number. I smiled and thought of Faith, picturing her "Jesus Loves Me" T-shirt. Faith had God's email and phone number. Now I did too.

In your yoga nidra practice, while you may not always enter turiya, the divine is always whispering to you. This is why you listen to your soul whisper every time you practice yoga nidra—to get the message. Yogi Desai also said, "Anything you create outside can be sold. If you create it inside, nobody can sell it." This is what I want for you.

Before Tanzania, I had been practicing yoga nidra for rest, because I was so sleep deprived, and it helped me feel well rested in my life. As a consequence, I was nicer to my children, husband, and so many others. I also had greater focus. But when I came back to yoga nidra after Tanzania, it was no longer just for rest. All those years ago, when I discovered yoga nidra at my local yoga studio, I thought that the twenty-five women I saw lying down were getting the best sleep of their lives—and they were. But I had no idea that the blissed-out looks on their faces also came from this deeper sense that everything in their lives was going to be okay. I may have experienced that sense because of yoga nidra before Tanzania, but after Tanzania, I had lost it. Difficult times in your life might do this, disrupt your connection with the divine. What I learned—and what you can learn too—is that if you are going through post-traumatic stress or any situation where you have lost hope, where you feel abandoned by the divine, that you can get it back. Yoga nidra helps you find your way back.

Knowing everything will be okay, and having God on speed dial, does not protect you from life falling apart. Instead, it provides a foundation for you to use to come back to that inner knowing and higher consciousness during difficult times. I hope for you, now, that foundation can be built with yoga nidra. It takes effort to rebuild your life from places that are broken, but when you succeed, the new structure you've built is much stronger and cannot easily be rebroken.

Optional: More Practices for Your Bliss Body

Here are a few practices to help balance your bliss body and complement your yoga nidra practice.

Activate Your Fourth Power Center

A balanced bliss body increases your ability to feel compassion and love for everything in your life. It is connected to the fourth power center, which is located in the center of the chest just above the heart. Don't get caught up in the bliss body being some fictitious place of perfection where you only feel huge amounts of joy. For many of us, feeling that everything will be okay is the first step to activating joy. To increase this vibration in your life, during days 26 through 30, consider putting your touchstone on your heart when you practice yoga nidra meditation. You might also like to use neroli essential oil on your clothing or rub it into your hands and inhale. An excellent color to wear to increase heart energy is pink or green.

Inhale Joy

Inhaling joy is a great practice to do when you're feeling a sense of alienation and lack of compassion for yourself and others. This is based on a beautiful part of the iRest yoga nidra meditation protocol. You can also do this practice at the end of yoga nidra meditation. Here's how you do it:

1. Remember a time when you felt joyful. It could be a very brief moment, like a memory of being with a favorite grandparent or seeing your child graduate.

2. Let your body feel that feeling of joy.

3. Let the memory fade and the feeling of joy remain. Take at least three or more slow breaths feeling joy.

4. Visualize joy spreading throughout your body. You might want to envision a smile starting in your heart and spreading through every nerve and cell of your body. Or see joy as a color and watch the color spread from your toes to the crown of your head. The point is to be absorbed in the feeling of joy.

5. Ask yourself: *If joy could speak, what would it say?* Ask for an image, word, or phrase.

6. Be curious about what you receive, but don't assign a story to it. Let it be.

Laugh

At the first yoga nidra meditation training I took, the class returned from lunch, and Richard Miller, the founder of iRest yoga nidra, began the next session by laughing. We all sat there looking at him—many of us smiling, waiting for him to stop—but he kept on laughing, straight from his belly, the sound carrying quite far. A minute or two later, others began laughing too. It took me a while, but after about five minutes, I could no longer resist, and I too started to laugh. At first it was a fake laugh, but soon, as if I caught the virus, I was laughing with full gusto. And while it was fun to laugh, here's the point: laughter can open your heart. Laughter helps you step out of your individuality and merge with the whole.

How to start? Go to a laughter yoga class. (Yes, there are such things.) Or get a group of friends or family members together; one of you starts laughing, and this will trigger others to laugh. This is a great activity to do with your entire family. You can even laugh by yourself in front of the mirror. Keep laughing for at least ten minutes.

Nurture Others

People often feel bliss when they're nurturing others. Notice I didn't say, "when they take care of others." While nurturing and caretaking are similar concepts, to me, nurturing comes from a place of choice, while caretaking feels like something you have to do.

One of the biggest lessons yoga nidra teaches us is that we have choices in how we approach a situation. If you are a caretaker (perhaps of parents, kids, or a loved one), it is essential to do as the airlines instruct: put your oxygen mask on first and then secure it on someone you are taking care of. This means to be sure you are nurturing yourself before you start nurturing others.

If you're not a caretaker, then nurturing others could mean volunteering at an animal shelter, a hospital, or a home for seniors; growing a garden to nurture plants; or helping a new mom with her baby.

Whatever form of nurturing you do, and whomever or whatever you nurture, the more you serve with love, the greater compassion you'll feel for all parts of your own life.

Optional: Diving Deeper

Looking to dive more deeply into your bliss, your authentic self, or sharing a difficult story? Consider these Daring to Rest optional prompts:

- Now that you have been practicing yoga nidra meditation for a while, what does bliss mean to you? Draw, freewrite, or create a movement piece to the meaning of bliss.

- Who are you on the inside? How has yoga nidra helped you discover your authentic self? Freewrite on this topic.

- Share a difficult story you have been holding in your heart. Where do you feel this story in your body? How has practicing yoga nidra helped you to let go of the hold the memory had on your mind and to see that everything will be all right? Freewrite on these questions or speak your answers into a recording device.

- If you have given birth or attended a birth, freewrite on the moment the baby was born. Give lots of details about how this event made you feel. After telling this story, how do you feel in your body? Freewrite again.

- Freewrite in your journal about your soul whispers.

Key Points in Chapter Nine

- Your bliss body is the fifth of five bodies of awareness that reside in you. It is the place that knows everything is going to be okay.

- It's here in the bliss body that you see your true self. When the bliss body is balanced, there are no more illusions surrounding you, and the final layer of emotional exhaustion dissolves.

- During yoga nidra meditation, you're being guided to the deepest state of consciousness, a fourth dimension known as turiya. Here you experience profound stillness, you are essentially thoughtless, and your unconscious mind is completely open to affirmations and intentions.

- It is in the bliss body that you find your internal power switch because the bliss body reveals the soul.

- In hard times, connecting to your bliss body via yoga nidra reminds you that everything is going to be okay.

Phase Three

RISE

When sleeping women wake, mountains move.

CHINESE PROVERB

After you've given attention to your five bodies, your vibrant, whole self becomes visible to you and often to others. This third phase of the Daring to Rest program is about rising up to lead from your most authentic self, and to dream big, which releases the final layer of exhaustion: life-purpose exhaustion.

Life-purpose exhaustion could mean that you're not in the right job or not pursuing your dreams. But it doesn't always mean you're not enjoying your life. Many women come into my rest programs feeling that they are in a job and life they love, but they just don't know how to manage their life without chronically burning out. In this final phase, you will take your yoga nidra "out of the bed" and learn how to use it to live a well-rested lifestyle. To do that, you'll first need to lead differently and dream big from this well-rested place.

Why is leading differently and rising up so important for women? To answer that question, it's important to understand women's complicated history with rest and how that history has held us back from our power. The truth is that our culture has tried to subdue women's wildish nature for centuries. From the mid-nineteenth century until the late 1910s, upper-middle-class women were routinely prescribed "rest cures" to help them recover from "nerves," "sick headaches," and other inexplicable ailments. Creative women received the strictest of rest cures, often being told not to get out of bed for fear they might write or do something irrational. "Innate feminine weakness" became a label attached to women, and even today we still see it applied to us.

Charlotte Perkins Gilman, a feminist writer in the late nineteenth century, was told by her doctor in 1887 to "live as domestic a life as far as possible" and "never to touch pen, brush or pencil again as long as I live," in addition to getting extensive bed rest.[1] In 1892 Gilman wrote the semiautobiographical short story "The Yellow Wallpaper," a fictional account through which she (indirectly) bashes the doctor who put her on the rest cure. Why? Because she knew that the rest cure was causing her creative spark to go out, and she suspected that might even be its underlying intention.

Women like Gilman didn't receive this prescription without a reason. Huge numbers of middle- and upper-middle-class women began showing signs of invalidism in the late 1800s, soon after the industrial revolution when women's roles became essentially restricted to organizing the household, having sex with their husbands, and raising children. Not surprisingly, they began to fall apart mentally. But how was the rest cure a solution? How could a woman like Gilman, who considered herself a writer, lie in bed, do nothing, and never write again? Gilman saw this as an assault on her entire being. Today, I'd call this an attempt to extinguish her Wild Woman.

In Gilman's time, rejecting rest was a good bargain. It helped women move forward, feed their wildish nature, and get out of bed and into the world. Today, there is a growing movement of women who are beginning to choose an even better bargain: we are embracing rest, and we're doing it on our own terms, journeying through programs like this, embracing a slower-paced life, tuning in to rhythm, and leading differently as a result. In the past, rest cures were prescribed to repress women's desires and inspiration and to keep them in a place of domestic subservience. Today, when we dare to rest, we are doing so to get back in touch with our desires and our inspiration because this feeds our Wild Woman. We are prescribing ourselves a new rest cure—one that says we are no longer subservient to modern society's dictum to "do more, be less."

Today's times need more brave women modeling rest; reclaiming a legitimate, healthy need for real relaxation; and leading from this well-rested place. Yes, there are real barriers in the workplace that don't support the realities of today's world, where women are caretakers in some capacity (for children, parents, pets) for most of their lives. Women like Arianna Huffington, with her "sleep revolution," are leading the cause to help address workplace barriers and shatter women's bad bargain with rest, showing us that we can dream big and rest—that it's not an either-or situation. There's still work to do, but like a pendulum, the groundswell of so many worn-out women in the world is beginning to turn the tide.

Our bad bargain with rest is a thread that runs deep. While it may feel convenient to blame cultural demands on women for our lack of rest, which certainly do exist, the root of overdoing is often tied to worthiness issues—not feeling worthy of love and success. The rising-up energy we'll explore in the final phase of our Daring to Rest journey is about how to live a lifestyle aligned with the five-bodies model you've just moved through, making sure you water all five bodies and demand a soul-driven life that asks, "What about me?" Your well-rested woman has been talking to you these past thirty days through your soul whispers; now it's time to act on what she's been saying and rise up.

Hopefully, by now, practicing yoga nidra has taught you that when you drop into the deepest state of consciousness, absolute stillness, you remember who you truly are. The challenge is to trust in who you are even when you're not practicing yoga nidra so that you don't lead from a place of who you are not. That was initially Gilman's problem—she was unable to be her authentic self in the real world where women's value seemed to not matter. Her turning point? Rejecting rest and becoming a writer, exactly what she was told not to do, but her authentic self said otherwise. It takes courage to stand in your authentic self, but now you're ready. Yoga nidra has prepared you for this moment to rise.

I always tell women that yoga nidra is an opportunity to lie down and wake up. You have already been "waking up" for thirty days to your authentic self and some big realizations about how your life has to change, but now you will begin to envision how to make these changes happen because living life asleep is exhausting. Gilman and other women in previous centuries fought to stay connected to the Wild Woman within them so that they could keep their internal power switches fully turned on, so that they could stay in their creative hot spots, and so that they could hear the intuitive voices that guide us to be who we are, not who we were told to be.

Gilman also fought to stay awake to her purpose in life because she saw this contributing to a world where more women were liberated from the chains of cultural expectations. When you are your truest self, you become the change you seek in the world—through your work, home life, and relationships—and this change ripples into the world. It doesn't matter if you stay at home with your children or you run a business—the formula is the same. This final phase is about asking, "Are my choices in harmony with me?" Because when you do what enlivens your soul, the final layer of exhaustion lifts.

My Kenyan friend Faith illustrated this point to me so beautifully when, years after the robbery, we were texting about a dream I have of setting up an academy that would teach women and girl leaders the Daring to Rest program. I told her I was concerned that so many young women in high school, college, and beyond are experiencing anxiety, depression, and sleep issues. Many of them are losing their confidence, zest for life, and desire to contribute to the world as leaders. I told Faith, "I want to make a difference." Here's her simple response: "Imagination is free. I am already praying for the academy."

As you move through these final ten days of the Daring to Rest program, I encourage you to remember Faith's words: "Imagination is free." This perhaps sums up the magic that yoga nidra infuses you with—permission to rest, permission to dream big again, and permission to lead from a well-rested place that expresses exactly who you are. It's now time to enter our final phase together, so hold on to your yoga nidra pompoms, dear Sister, and here we go.

10

LEAD

A New Model of Embracing All of You

Days 31–35

The beauty of yoga nidra is that after cleaning up your five bodies while consciously sleeping, you are pointed back to your true nature, and this juicy spot, where you are unapologetically you, is the ideal place to lead from. This is the well-rested woman—calm, wild, and free to be herself.

For centuries, our wildness has been locked up and vilified. In the 1900s, a woman who was viewed as falling apart mentally might receive an ovariectomy, removal of the ovaries, as an estimated 150,000 women did because it was believed that the ovaries controlled a woman's personality. Sounds insane now, but this is one way society has tried to control our Wild Woman. This control has led us to doubt our true selves and send our true natures into hiding. Well, no more. When you're practicing yoga nidra, you can't hide because each time you lie down, you feel who you are in every cell in your body. Yoga nidra helps us know ourselves deeply, feel confident, and of course, get the deep rest we need to shine.

When you have embraced who you truly are, you are able to model a new, feminine style of leadership. This is whole-person leadership. Most women accomplish more when they lead from their whole, truest selves, and they're happier too. Modeling feminine leadership is the key to staying well rested, and changing the world.

A few years ago I attended a workshop by Tara Brach, an inspiring meditation teacher, therapist, and well-known author. She explained that the purpose of meditation was not to find your goals in life, but rather your "gold." That's what we've been doing with yoga nidra: daring to rest for gold, not goals. Now it's time to take what you've learned through your yoga nidra meditation—your gold—and use it to bring purpose and power to how you lead your life and to realize your big dreams.

Basic Instructions for Days 31 to 35

1. Practice the Phase Three: Rise Meditation daily. Continue to use your most recent intention and your touchstone. You might like to place your touchstone on your throat to activate the fifth power center or on the space between your eyebrows to activate the sixth power center.

2. At the end of yoga nidra, listen for and track your soul whispers.

3. Optional: Continue to practice connecting with your Council of Women outside of your yoga nidra meditation.

4. Optional: Discover your big dreams and start using a big dream as your intention during yoga nidra meditation if it feels right.

5. Optional: Use additional practices to help you lead from a place of embracing all of yourself.

6. Optional: Use the Diving Deeper prompts to explore obstacles to well-rested leadership and use storytelling to envision and embrace your well-rested woman.

Feminine Leadership Keeps Us Well Rested

As you've seen over the last thirty days, cleaning each body of awareness lead us to our soul, the seat of wholeness:

The physical body: Deep rest, safety, groundedness

The energy body: Life force, vitality, rhythm

The mental body: Transforming the mind, greeting emotions

The wisdom body: Intuition, the Wild Woman, self-trust, consciousness

The bliss body: Spiritual connectedness, freedom from suffering, life-purpose connection

If you're feeling worn out, at least one of these bodies is not balanced. The good news is that in addition to yoga nidra, you now have many other practices—a whole Daring to Rest toolbox—to help you keep all five bodies clear and balanced, all of which support a well-rested lifestyle. "Well-rested" doesn't mean that you're never tired; instead, it means you have the tools you need to nourish your wholeness and stay connected to your Wild Woman. This, in turn, will help you in difficult situations or when you need to make tough decisions, and will make it easier to recover from difficulty and focus again on the things that matter to you.

Pacing yourself, focusing on rhythm—and on the things that matter deeply to you—is feminine leadership. I've seen again and again how embracing it can radically change women's levels of exhaustion. It helps them step out of leading with more masculine traits like doing, planning, achieving, and organizing. Feminine leadership leads with what I call the "slow down, feel, then act" model of leadership: it promotes slowing down, receiving, and then acting from a place of fullness. A well-rested woman leads from a feminine leadership model like the five-bodies model, because it supports her wholeness, and this wholeness supports her ability to lead.

The Truth about Feminine Leadership

Feminine leadership has nothing to do with gender; instead, it is a style of leading rooted in empathy, communication, and consciousness. It's about bringing your whole self to everything you lead, whether it's at work or at home. Right now, the world is starved for feminine leadership. This kind of leadership, which both women and men can embrace, is about leading with awareness.

Many people perceive feminine leadership to be weak leadership. I would argue that it's not weak at all: this is leadership with lots of awareness, intuition, and strong boundaries. Is it different from the paradigm many of us are living in now? Yes. It is rooted in the knowledge that everything is going to be okay. And when it's not okay, that doesn't mean you have to go into fear or attack mode. You can acknowledge a difficult moment and recognize that it will pass. Yoga nidra meditation teaches us, in every body of awareness, that meeting a sensation deactivates its charge and its effect on you.

Feminine leadership is leading from the heart and feelings. As ALisa Starkweather, founder of the Red Tent Temple Movement for women, posted on her Facebook page, feeling an emotion like sadness "is not to be confused with despair, or giving up, or weakness or defeat but rather a testament of engagement with deep caring, kindness, love and the willingness to keep my eyes wide open."[1] Feminine leadership, just like yoga nidra, is an awakened state. It allows you to be authentic and not fall into the female psychic slumber mentioned in chapter one. As ALisa said, feeling all of her emotions helps her take a stand and show up to lead. Women have denied this side of ourselves for too long, and we've especially shied away from expressing it through our leadership. In order to be "good girls," we've accepted a way of leading that's not in alignment with balance and wholeness. Hopefully, yoga nidra has taught you that if you start with feeling, then the warrior, a more masculine energy, will also rise, but it will rise out of a deeply sacred feminine space. We need more leaders who lead from a peaceful, heart-based model because that's the energy that spreads peace.

Being and Becoming

Once you find yoga nidra, it's tempting to use it only for deep rest—nourishment of the body. The problem is that eventually your soul says that you also need to live your purpose. Rebooting your energy requires a fully charged body and soul. The Vedic teachings, a source of yoga science and philosophy, inform us that our soul needs both being and becoming. We tend to think of the soul as this calm state of being that wants nothing. There is actually another aspect of the soul that calls you to live your purpose.

In some ways, being and becoming seem contradictory because if you need nothing and reside in a state of just being, then desires or your unique destiny shouldn't matter. But the soul reveals that both coexist: you are both stillness and striving. People who burn out forget this and embrace only the striving. I believe this is why meditation is so popular—our culture is craving a state of being to balance all the striving.

The problem we face is how to determine what our soul desires, so we don't just grab every desire out there. If we followed all the strivings of the mind, we'd sit and eat chocolate cake, date the best-looking person who walks in the door, or starve ourselves to look fabulous for that good-looking person. Listening to your soul whispers for the past thirty days has prepared you to not grab at those ego-driven desires. All leaders listen to soul whispers in some way, if not through yoga nidra, then by building regular quiet time into their lives in some other way. This helps them discover their gold and lead from it.

Mining Your Gold for Big Dreams

I love the word *gold* for the lessons we learn through yoga nidra because I immediately think of the hero's journey, a pattern of storytelling followed by many fairy tales, books, and films and explored by Joseph Campbell in his book *The Hero with a Thousand Faces*. Dorothy's journey in *The Wizard of Oz* is an example of a hero's journey. According to Campbell, a hero goes on a journey that includes the following steps:

1. She's living her ordinary life.

2. She gets called to an adventure that will change her life.

3. She meets a mentor to help her get through the adventure.

4. She experiences many trials during the adventure, and together these act as an initiation to change her life.

5. She survives the adventure and finds the gold.

6. She returns home with the gold.

The hero's journey of a woman following the Daring to Rest program is very similar:

1. She begins the journey asleep (living a busy, stressed-out life).

2. She gets called to wake up (by experiencing burnout, illness, or some crisis).

3. She resists the call (keeps staying too busy).

4. She finally succumbs to the adventure of waking up physically, mentally, and emotionally (via the physical body, energy body, and mental body). This may present challenges and dark moments, but it also prompts her to change her life.

5. She then experiences an awakening (via the wisdom body and bliss body, often through telling or remembering an untold story).

6. She finds victory—the gold (her internal power switch, her true self).

7. She returns to her life to share the gold (to dream big).

This is the journey you have been on. Now you're in the final stretch, ready to reflect on the gold you've found, bring it into your everyday life, and share it. It's time to look at the soul whispers you've gathered over the past thirty days and see what big dreams lie in their messages.

One woman came into my rest program having lost a child nearly ten years earlier. When she reviewed her soul whispers after thirty days, she felt her child's voice kept coming through. One soul whisper was, "I'm okay, Mommy." Another was, "Go for it." By day 30, it was clear to her that her gold, the lesson she learned, was that "I am strong"—something she hadn't felt since her son's death. She knew immediately what this lesson meant: it was time to turn a devastating situation into something better. Her big dream? She started a local food and toy bank for families because her son had always loved helping homeless families during the holidays. Sometimes after resting for forty days, our big dreams are crystal clear to us, as they were for this woman; other times they're less so. But all big dreams are powerful and often lead to taking inspired action, a combination of head- and heart-based action.

Valerie Estelle Frankel, a professor, storyteller, and author, tells us that women experience the hero's journey with a feminine twist: "While the hero journeys for external fame, fortune, and power, the heroine tries to regain her lost creative spirit. . . . Once she hears the cries of this lost part of herself needing rescue, her journey truly begins."[2] This lost creative spirit that you found during your Daring to Rest journey is your gold, the lesson you learned. For the woman in my rest program who lost her child, her gold was rediscovering "I am strong." Other women in my rest programs have found that their gold is to know "I am enough," "I am worthy," "I am sexual," "I am woman," "I am beautiful," "I am safe," or "I am sacred." These are the parts of their creative spirit that they rediscovered from their Daring to Rest journey and took back into everyday life.

What part of your lost creative spirit are you taking back? At the beginning of the Daring to Rest program, the answer would most likely have come from your head. Your gold always comes from your heart and soul, and your big dreams do too.

If "I am enough" is your gold, this might mean one of your big dreams is ending a lifelong eating disorder. If "I am safe" is your gold, this could mean fulfilling a dream of volunteering at a rape crisis center or even starting your own organization to support women survivors of rape and sexual assault. Your gold often resembles an intention statement. For Margreet, her "I am safe" intention was also her gold, as it gave her the permission to open her own business despite years of not trusting herself because of a difficult childhood. How did she know it was her gold? Because it came up in her soul whispers, and she felt it as a guiding light as she practiced yoga nidra meditation for many continuous days.

Four Steps for Discovering Your Big Dreams

Here is a four-step process for discovering your big dreams within your gold. As you go through this process on days 31 to 35, try to do it without focusing on an outcome; focus more on how you can feel whole and birth who you are, your true nature, into everything you do. After choosing one big dream, you may choose to use this to create a new intention statement to use as you continue your yoga nidra meditations.

Step One: Create a Soul Whispers Board or Book

On days 31 to 33, use the words and images of your soul whispers from days 1 through 30 to create a soul whispers board. Use a sheet of poster board and glue the words and images from your soul whispers on it. Another option is to create a soul whispers book. Use separate pieces of paper to express each soul whisper on its own page. Punch holes in the pages to tie them together. (You can untie the pages and add additional soul whispers for these last ten days of your journey.)

Practice the Phase Three: Rise Meditation before you work on your soul whispers board or book each day.

Step Two: Create Your Gold Statement

On day 34, practice the Phase Three: Rise Meditation with your soul whispers board or book placed near the top of your head.

After the yoga nidra meditation, put your left hand over your heart, look at all the words and images on your soul whispers board or book, and notice how you feel in your body. Then ask for a song that sums up these soul whispers. You may hear the title of the song, or you may hear lyrics from the song. This song should feel like your theme song at this moment, a positive song that represents the true you. This song title or lyric is your gold statement, summing up the lessons you've received during your first thirty days.

On a new sheet of paper or another poster board, draw a tree and write your gold statement (the song's name or lyrics) on the trunk of the tree. If you hear nothing when you ask for a song, write "I feel" on the tree trunk.

Step Three: Create Your Big Dream Statement(s)

Take a deep breath and read your gold statement. Put your hand over your heart, take a slow, deep breath in through your heart, and say to yourself: "Knowing my gold is (state your gold statement), my big dream is . . ." Then pause. What do you hear? Write what you receive—no more than one sentence—on a branch growing out of your tree. You can ask for up to three big dreams, if you wish, or stick with one.

Write each big dream you receive on a branch of your tree. Each branch is a big dream for the coming year. Make sure each big dream aligns with your gold statement. Each big dream statement must be positive, concise, and from your heart, not your head.

Step Four: Choose One Big Dream

On day 35, practice the Phase Three: Rise Meditation and, immediately afterward, read your big dream(s) for this year. Then close your eyes and imagine your Council of Women appearing. Put your hand over your heart, close your eyes, and breathe in through your heart. If you have more than one big dream, ask them, "Where do I start? Which big dream should I follow?" If you have a single big dream, simply ask, "Where do I start?"

Listen to their answers. Don't overthink this. Notice what dream you're guided to start with or what first step you're guided to take. Pass it through your gut and heart. Does it feel true to you? If so, begin using this big dream statement as the intention for your yoga nidra mediations through the completion of the forty days (and beyond, if that feels right).

*

The key to moving through all four steps is to trust your intuition—that's your Wild Woman nature. Remember, you're practicing a feminine model of operating: slow down, feel, and then act.

Judith had spent years working as a busy doula but feeling as though she wasn't being heard, recognized, or successful. Cancer was her wake-up call. Two years after going through chemotherapy and radiation, Judith was ready to embrace a new way of being and thrive. After practicing yoga nidra, she very quickly discovered her gold from her soul whispers: "I am wise, wild, and willow." From this gold statement, she got three big dreams, one for each word in her gold statement.

> *Wise*: "I am writing a memoir that introduces an
> evolutionary meme to the cancer culture."

> *Wild*: "I nourish, invigorate, strengthen, and oxygenate
> all cell tissues through daily movement (dance, music,
> yoga, walking, biking)."

> *Willow*: "I am breathing and tuning in, deepening
> a clearer communication with divine guidance, and
> learning to be more flexible in life and flow through
> winds of adversity."

Your big dreams may not be directly related to the words in your gold statement, like Judith's were, but they should always be aligned with your gold statement.

Discovering your big dreams requires you to remember that the path to well-rested is imperfect. Your dreams may not come true, but your gold is perennial. If your big dream does not manifest the way you expected, this does not mean that yoga nidra is not working for you. The path may not look familiar or be the one you thought you were taking, but keep your eyes open—your dreams don't always bloom into the color you expect.

Optional: Practices to Help You Lead as a Well-Rested Woman

Leading your life as a well-rested woman may be a completely new way of operating for you, so remember to be gentle and kind to yourself. You're learning to live and work more in a receiving mode. Following are practices to help you receive in order to lead.

Activate the Fifth and Sixth Power Centers

Days 31 through 35 are a great time to activate the fifth and sixth power centers. These power centers are important for dreaming big. The fifth power center is located in the throat area and helps you speak your truth and listen from your higher self. The sixth power center is located at the third eye, the space between the eyebrows on the forehead, and helps you see beyond the boundaries of right and wrong. You might like to put your touchstone on your throat to activate the fifth power center or on the space between your eyebrows to activate the sixth power center. Any stimulating essential oil, like peppermint, is good for activating rising-up energy. For the fifth power center, a great color to wear is blue. For the sixth power center, wear indigo.

Anointing Practice for the Rise Phase

Here's another essential oil practice from Deborah Sullivan to do after your yoga nidra meditation any time during the Rise phase (days 31 to 40).

Choose an essential oil that feels empowering, such as vetiver or ginger, and apply it to your forehead, heart, and belly. Feel this oil as an initiation or consecration of the Wild Woman rising up in your body and your soul. Read the following words into a recording device, if desired.

> As you anoint your forehead, heart, and belly, you invoke the ancestral ways that are transmitted through the elements, the primal forces of Mother Nature and the unseen realms. The three power centers associated with these parts of the body are sacred receptacles, holy vessels through which spirit can manifest in creation. Your forehead is for wisdom and intuition, your heart is for compassion and unconditional love, and your belly is for creative power and taking sacred action.
>
> Feel the alignment of these three energies rising up in your mind, heart, and body. Sense the comingling of these attributes pulsing through your body and beyond your body as the scent surrounds you.
>
> Now imagine a golden bubble around your body glowing with luminosity. Envision a way of walking on your soul path that reflects the energies of these three scared centers working in perfect balance and harmony.
>
> Listen to any messages, images, or visions that may be rising up as you embody your wholeness, as you remember the untamed nature of the Wild Woman that is emerging through you and as you.
>
> Just sit in the silence and stillness, feel a spacious field of love, peace, and beauty all around you. Be a conduit for the energies of light, love, and beauty united within and all around you, radiating out in all directions for the next seven generations and beyond as a blessing.

Practice Sensing and Saying Yes and No

One of the most exhausting stress loops for women starts with saying yes when we feel no. The problem is that the worn-out woman doesn't know what a yes and no feels like in her body. We often tell women to say no more, but equally troublesome is that we also don't feel and then follow our yeses.

Here's a quick way to practice sensing what yes and no feel like to you:

1. Put one hand on your heart and one on your gut.

2. Place your attention at the space between your eyebrows (your third eye).

3. Take three breaths using the *So Hum* Breath from chapter eight. Inhale from the space between your eyebrows to the base of your spine while mentally saying the sound *Soooooo*. Then exhale from the base of your spine to the space between your eyebrows while mentally saying the sound *Hummmmmm*.

4. Be still as you rest your attention on your third eye for twenty to thirty seconds.

5. Call up a question you want an answer to and see if you feel a yes or no.

For women who have lots of decisions to make, like mothers, I often suggest making a list of all the things stressing them out, and then, on the same day every week, doing this practice, seeing if they get a yes or no for each item on the list. This is also a great practice to do weekly when you're pregnant because giving birth centered in your true self, knowing your yes and no, is the best gift you can give your baby. If you have extra time, practice yoga nidra first and then do this practice.

Using this practice to help make decisions will help you stop over-doing. You begin with feeling, drop your ego, and then, from your true nature, make decisions that end the worn-out feeling. Beware of mistaking things you love to do as a yes. For example, many of the creative moms I work with love to cook, but when they use this practice to ask whether they want to stay up baking cupcakes late at night for their children's school when they have work the next day, the answer they get might well be no.

Sometimes you may be faced with a difficult no: your inner wisdom will tell you that saying no to something will liberate time, but saying no may not feel good right away or may disappoint someone. If this happens, I encourage you to say no anyway. If you want to feel well-rested, you need to make the hard choices that support your wholeness.

Love Yourself First

The first thing your loved ones need is a healthy you. Here are two ways to help you put yourself first, then others.

Give kindness. When you're spinning in mental loops, stressed out, it's hard to be kind to yourself or others. But as I always say, after yoga nidra, I feel like I drank a cup of kindness. To capitalize on and reinforce this feeling after you practice yoga nidra, sit up and repeat this lovingkindness meditation to yourself:

> May I be happy.
> May I be safe.
> May I be free of physical pain and suffering.
> May I be able to recognize and touch harmony and joy
> in myself.
> May I nourish wholesome seeds in myself.
> May I be healthy, peaceful, and strong.

Notice how you feel in your body. When you're ready, you can move on to saying the words for others: *May (name of a loved one) be happy. May (he/she) be safe.*

Go on wonder dates. Schedule quiet time for yourself. My friend and colleague Jeffrey Davis, of the creative branding company Tracking Wonder, loves to say, "Wonder is not kid's stuff. It's radical grown-up stuff." That's right—taking time for wonder is an essential multivitamin for adults too. It helps clear your mind and relax the body.

What's wonder? It's a time to be curious, to not know something. It's the gratitude and amazement we feel when we see a shooting star or a beautiful full moon. Try finding a quiet space to read poetry, or sit in a tree and then journal about what you see and how it makes you feel. Many spots in nature call up wonder. Wonder sparks ideas, so the more time you spend in wonder, the juicier you will feel when you return to your everyday life.

And if you think you don't have time, think again. Jeffrey has two little girls, and as he says, he "sculpts time" for wonder by intentionally scheduling it in his calendar.

Optional: Diving Deeper

Looking to dive more deeply into embracing your well-rested woman? Consider these Daring to Rest optional prompts:

- What's gotten in the way of you leading in any area of your life in the past? Why? What have you learned from practicing yoga nidra to help you lead differently now? Freewrite on this topic.

- Write your worn-out woman's story. Who is she? How and why was she overdoing? Be vulnerable. Explore issues of worthiness. Then write your well-rested woman's story. Who is she? How and why is she giving herself permission to rest? If you don't feel the well-rested woman's story yet in your life, imagine it and write it as a fairy tale with you as the protagonist. If you wish, dance or draw these two stories instead of writing them.

- Write or act out a scene of your well-rested woman coaching your worn-out woman. Share lots of details, including what they're saying to each other, where

they're meeting, their body language, and what they're
wearing. At the end, notice how you feel in your body.

- Freewrite in your journal about your soul whispers.

- Look at the five bodies and the qualities you'll feel
  when they are balanced (located at the beginning of
  this chapter). Identify a body you need to focus on
  balancing. Why? What steps can you take to balance it?

Key Points in Chapter Ten

- Well-rested women own their Wild Woman—their intuition,
  awareness, and sensitivity—and lead from this place.

- Our soul needs both *being* and *becoming*. Well-
  rested women feed both sides of themselves.

- Model feminine leadership by leading from
  empathy, emotions, rhythm, and consciousness.

- The purpose of meditation, including yoga nidra, is
  to find your gold, not goals. Your gold is the lost part
  of you that you rediscover when you go on a journey of
  self-discovery, like your Daring to Rest journey.

- Your gold helps you discover your big dreams in life. Your
  big dreams may involve an outcome, but like an intention,
  they still are an expression of your true nature.

11

LIFE

Daring to Rest Forever

Days 36–40

For these final five days of the Daring to Rest program, the focus is bringing together all the principles you've learned to help you envision deep rest as a lifestyle. Instead of complaining about what doesn't work, a well-rested woman creates the lifestyle that does work for her. You now have the yoga nidra road map. Of course, you'll be tempted to fall back into the worn-out woman spin because the hypnotic pull of our culture has trained us to hide our true selves, accepting norms that feel unacceptable in our bones, for a long time. But now you know that your health and well-being depend on you not following the worn-out woman model. This is what's been expected of you, and it's not working. It's time to create the life that's right for you—not a perfect life, but one that includes daring to rest.

Basic Instructions for Days 36 to 40

1. Practice the Phase Three: Rise Meditation daily, using your big dream statement as your intention. Continue to use this intention until a new intention makes itself known during your yoga nidra or through your soul whispers.

2. Continue to listen for and track your soul whispers at the end of yoga nidra. This is forever medicine.

3. Optional: Continue to practice connecting with your Council of Women outside of your yoga nidra meditation.

4. Optional: Use additional practices to check in to see how rested you are and to make use of your touchstone.

5. Optional: Use the Diving Deeper prompts to reflect on your Daring to Rest journey, envision your well-rested self, create a plan to practice yoga nidra in the future, and explore who to share it with.

Daring to Rest Principles to Live By

While I've taught you about yoga nidra meditation in a linear way, using the trinity of rest, release, and rise and the five-bodies model as our map, you can expect to circle in and out of each phase again and again, depending on where you are in your life. Following are some concepts within each phase that can act as guiding principles for your new, well-rested woman.

Lead from your heart. Yoga nidra always invites you, through body sensing and breath, to connect with your heart. When we disconnect from our hearts, we lose our connections to our souls. Soul whispers are your compass back to your heart and soul. Whenever you're feeling directionless, spend a week listening to your soul whispers, during or after yoga nidra, and then see what messages rise from that to steer you to a better place.

Meet darkness. When we shine consciousness on the shadow parts of ourselves, we exercise our bravery muscle. Meeting and greeting emotions or thoughts that feel dark is some of the healthiest release work we can do. Meeting darkness reveals the light. Yoga nidra teaches us that what we meet, we can safely go beyond. When you meet an emotion or thought during yoga nidra, this creates the potential to defuse the hold it has on you, and this permeates all parts of your life. Bottom line: Make friends with the dark.

Welcome everything just as it is. Resist the cultural tidal wave trying to pull you into separateness and into thinking of your life and the world as an either-or dichotomy; persist in believing in a both-and way of thinking. Jungian feminist psychologist Marion Woodman tells us that wholeness comes from "holding the tension of the opposites."[1] Allow yourself to feel the discomfort of holding everything and changing nothing. Yoga nidra teaches us how to do this when we hold opposites. In chapter seven, you learned how to use Holding Opposites in your everyday life too. Use it often and everywhere—during family dinners, at work, when you're feeling pain during menstruation, and while giving birth, when you think you can't, but know you can. It will help you feel free from the exhausting mental loop.

You are always supported. Yoga nidra connects you to a universal feeling of oneness. It's here that you realize the universe always has your back. As extra assurance, and to help you take this support into your everyday life, be sure to call up your Council of Women. After you have been calling them up regularly in your yoga nidra practice, you will be able to more readily call on them as support outside of yoga nidra, at times in your life when you feel you need mentorship or guides. These wise women guides always see you for who you truly are, and this helps you see your true nature.

Unleash your Wild Woman. Your Wild Woman, the highly intuitive woman who carries and honors the stories of your outer and inner worlds, is always there; you just have to stop and listen for her. Spending time in your inner world, using practices like yoga nidra meditation or sitting in nature, will call your wildish nature forward. You need your Wild Woman fully turned on in order to lead.

Everything will be okay. It's easy to fall into darkness when we hit rough patches in life. But in the depths of yoga nidra, at the deepest state of consciousness, we are reminded that everything will be okay. We become grateful. We even touch into joy. Have trust and faith in your everyday life that the divine is always listening and whispering to you that everything will be okay. *You've got this.*

Telling a difficult story will set you free. There are portals to our souls, and telling a difficult story that you're holding is one of them. Clarissa Pinkola Estés says, "Stories . . . bring us news of just what to do about the women's wound that will not cease its bleeding."[2] Storytelling in a safe setting is a beautiful way to explore your wounds and stop the drain they have on your energy. Listening to the voice of your soul, through your soul whispers, clarifies the truth and gives you the bravery to tell a difficult story.

Imagination is free. One of the first childlike traits to leave adults is imagination. Adults have responsibilities, and often it feels like responsibility sabotages our ability to imagine our lives any differently. If my friend Faith can still believe in imagination, so can you. The only person stopping you from imagining yourself healthy, whole, and complete is you. In addition to yoga nidra, many of the freewriting practices in "Phase Three: Rise" are excellent for helping you free your imagination.

Stand in your authentic self. Feminine leadership thrives when women are leading from their authentic selves. Forget who everybody tells you to be. Be you. If you don't like a model that's out there in society, create a new model. This includes everything from executive leadership to teaching to parenting. The more you stand in your truest self, the more you feel whole. Yoga nidra is a pointer back to your authentic self, so whenever you feel you're not sure who you are, lie down, practice yoga nidra, and listen to your soul whispers. You may also want to give attention to whichever of the five bodies needs watering by practicing some of the optional tools in that body's corresponding chapter.

Serve you first, then others. I end every yoga nidra meditation with the words "be good to yourself" because if there is a single lesson the Daring to Rest program teaches you, it's how to be good to yourself. This lesson is for life. It's the lesson of receiving, something women entering my rest programs have a hard time doing but desperately need to do. Yes, we can and must give, but we also must receive. The moment you understand this, you break from the long history of women serving from an exhausted place and begin to serve from a place of abundance. Yoga nidra is the tool to teach you this, again and again, until it becomes second nature.

Stay awake. Yoga nidra will help you wake up in your life, but staying awake takes consciousness of both the big and small things in your daily life. Notice how in rhythm you feel in your life, and when you're needing to go inward and make time for it—demand it. A nurtured inner world is essential for women and helps balance our outer world. Without our inner world, we fall asleep, wandering through life not fully engaged. All the practices in this book help you stay awake. An awakened woman is a well-rested woman.

How Much Yoga Nidra Meditation Do You Need Now?

Many women who have gone through the Daring to Rest program like to continue practicing yoga nidra daily. It just feels right because yoga nidra and rest have become a part of their lives. Now that you have a yoga nidra meditation practice, it doesn't matter how often you practice; what matters is how consistently you practice. Even if it's once per week, make that your nonnegotiable time to practice yoga nidra meditation.

In times of crisis, you may need a full day or a weekend of what I call Daring to Rest cave time to get you back on track. During this time, you'll take yourself through an abbreviated version of the Daring to Rest program. Begin by doing the fifteen-minute Phase One: Rest Meditation, and then you might choose to do a few optional practices from the phase one chapters. Freewriting in your journal about your soul whispers is my favorite optional practice because it's easy, powerful, and reveals very quickly how in or out of rhythm you feel. Then practice the thirty-minute Phase Two: Release Meditation and a few optional practices from phase two. And finally, end your day or weekend with a long, forty-minute Phase Three: Rise Meditation and maybe an optional practice from phase three. Remember to listen for soul whispers and use your touchstone throughout.

You might like to take an approach that considers the five-bodies model. Think about which particular body needs attention. For example, if you want to turn around negative thoughts, then you might want to focus on the mental body, practicing the Phase Two: Release Meditation and complementary practices in chapter seven. If you sense a disconnect from hope, then use the Phase Two: Release Meditation and focus on the bliss body to regain a connection to spirit. If you feel your heart needs attention, perhaps because you've been hurt and are unable to forgive someone, focus on the optional practices for the wisdom body. If you've not been resting much or feel your vitality is low, focus on the Phase One: Rest Meditation and nurture yourself with optional practices for the physical and energy bodies. You determine how long you focus on a specific body, but often either a twenty-one-day or forty-day practice in that one body is an ideal amount of time to feel a shift.

You might need yoga nidra daily. Caretakers such as postpartum moms and people like nurses, who are also shift workers, often need daily yoga nidra. The Phase One: Rest Meditation is excellent to use during these times, as are any optional practices for the physical and energy bodies in chapters five and six. It may seem impossible to practice every day; often people who practice daily do so in the morning, before they get out of bed, or in the evening, at bedtime. Eventually, practicing yoga nidra becomes as routine as brushing your teeth.

Menstruation is another important time to practice yoga nidra meditation more often, especially because hormone fluctuations can affect our sleep. This could mean doing just fifteen minutes of yoga nidra meditation daily and tracking your soul whispers every day during your menstruation. Or you may want to not practice daily, but commit to long yoga nidra naps on weekends when you have more time. You may wish to add some of the optional practices in this book on weekends. Women are particularly creative and "juicy" during their menstruation. If your flow is heavy, long yoga nidra meditations are useful, and freewriting in your journal about your soul whispers is essential because they will give you insight into the meaning behind the heavy flow. Also, you may wish to set an intention that you use just during your menstruation, to address heavy flow or discomfort.

If you're pregnant, you will have a dramatic change in your birth experience if you practice yoga nidra daily. If you are just starting your pregnancy, you could go through the Daring to Rest program three times, once in each trimester. Or you could go through the Daring to Rest program once and then continue practicing the shorter Phase One: Rest Meditation daily because pregnant moms need lots of rest. You could also continue practicing the longer yoga nidra meditations regularly until you give birth. Optional practices in the mental body chapter (chapter seven) are particularly useful during pregnancy—especially the Holding Opposites practice because it will help you manage emotions that may come up during the birth.

Also, you can practice yoga nidra meditation in the early stages of giving birth. Lots of women listen to yoga nidra meditation at this time; and as I mentioned in chapter seven, pregnant moms tell me it's deeply relaxing and helps them hold both the fear of giving birth and the deep knowing that they can give birth. You can use a yoga nidra meditation from any phase, but in your third trimester, the Phase Three: Rise Meditation is excellent because, with birth, you want to be relaxed but hold rising energy. Then, in the late stages of labor, you can use any of the breathing practices from the program or get up and move your body to get your life force flowing. During birth, the practices for the energy body in chapter six, and particularly for activating the second power center, will be useful. And you'll want to keep using the Holding Opposites practice because it helps you to hold intense emotions and thoughts and to disidentify with them, allowing you to come into a place of stillness, which is an ideal place for pushing a baby out. (Don't worry, you'll still have lots of warrior energy to push the baby out.)

If you're postpartum, when you truly have little time and are often up in the middle of the night, consider staying in the Rest phase for the first year or more. A consistent fifteen minutes of yoga nidra and listening to your soul whispers will make a huge difference and help balance all the activation with "rest-and-digest" energy. Many new moms I support will practice yoga nidra for fifteen minutes when the baby naps or just before bedtime. If you don't practice daily, then at least consider right after birth dedicating yourself to a forty-day period of yoga nidra. In Latin America, a custom called *la cuarentena* ("the quarantine") allows mothers forty days to recover from birth, bond with their baby, and rest. Makes sense, right?

For women in menopause who no longer bleed or who bleed irregularly, I suggest making a monthly Daring to Rest date in accordance with the full moon. Tune in to your deepest need to determine what phase you're in (Rest, Release, or Rise), and use the yoga nidra meditation for that phase. (For guidance, see "Assess How Rested You Are" later in this chapter.) Remember, all yoga nidra practices are restful, so you're tuning in to your *deepest* need, not just the surface need for rest. If you have a hard time choosing a phase, create guidance cards. On the full moon, write *rest*, *release*, and *rise* on three pieces of paper. Place all three pieces of paper face down, take a deep breath, and pick one with your left hand. Then practice the yoga nidra meditation for the phase you've picked. If you have time, also do one or two optional practices from that phase.

You can also choose to take one full day every month, like a spa day, and practice all three meditations. The days of the full moon and new moon are excellent days to choose. Full-moon energy helps us let go, as it symbolizes endings and completions, and new-moon energy symbolizes new beginnings and starting anew. One full day devoted to Daring to Rest is enough time to complete the following steps:

1. Practice yoga nidra meditation for the Rest phase.

2. Do one of the optional practices from the Rest phase.

3. Take a break to drink and eat something healthy.

4. Repeat steps 1 and 2 using the yoga nidra meditations and optional practices from the Release and Rise phases, with meal breaks in between.

Ultimately, you are the one who knows how much yoga nidra meditation you need and what Daring to Rest practices you want to use to supplement the meditations. Please, don't overthink this. In fact, many times in a live class, I will lay out laminated cards with all the Daring to Rest tools (see appendix 2) and encourage women to place them face down, breathe, and then with their left hands, pick a card. Then this is the Daring to Rest tool they practice after yoga nidra meditation. And guess what? They always receive the tool they need. You can do this too by writing the name of each tool/practice on an index card, turning the cards face down, and then picking a card. Simple, easy, and restful.

Share Yoga Nidra with Others

For many years, my husband worked for Heifer International, a charity committed to ending hunger and poverty. Most people know Heifer because of its catalog, which lists a variety of animals—like cows, goats, and chickens—you can choose to give to someone in a poor country. Then the people who receive the animal commit to "passing on the gift." For example, when their cow has a calf, they pass that calf along to someone else in their village. I love this concept and think about it a lot with yoga nidra meditation because now that you have this gift, you have a responsibility to pass on the gift to others. Doing so fully completes your Daring to Rest journey.

Passing on the Daring to Rest gift looks different for everyone. You may feel inspired to become trained to teach this program to others, or you may want to invite a friend or family member to dare to rest with you.

Sharing yoga nidra is a beautiful way to spread love. I consider couples yoga nidra meditation the best therapy ever. You and your partner wake up feeling kind and gentle toward each other. All the hard-line positions you argued about that day or that week fall away. It's like rebooting your relationship from zero. Family yoga nidra night is also delicious—a great way to come together and train your kids early to appreciate rest.

You may also want to get a partner or group of women and go through the Daring to Rest program together. Just like doing a yearly gut cleanse, planning to practice the Daring to Rest program yearly or even quarterly, with the seasons, will help you feel well rested and spread the yoga nidra magic to others. Gather your friends or neighbors to do it together.

I know men need yoga nidra meditation too. Men feel worn out in their bodies because of busy days and tiring messages like "man up" and "nice guys finish last." Many men have been raised in ways that do not feed their feminine desire to receive and show love. Many mothers today, myself included, are trying to change this as we raise our boys. But most men know only their masculine side because this is what our culture appreciates in men. Yoga nidra meditation is clearly needed in the workplace for both men and women. We women cannot change our culture and how women have been treated for centuries without healthy and peaceful men by our sides. More and more men want to change the culture too, and they want to feel more peace; they just don't have the skills and language to do so yet. Inviting them to lie down and practice yoga nidra meditation, so they can feel peace, is a start. Please, if there's a man in your life, even a neighbor who's suffering, introduce him to yoga nidra meditation.

Yoga nidra is also an opportunity for you to connect deeply and feel with another person, something that is much needed in our "do it alone" culture. When Sarah, from one of my yoga nidra programs, spent a weekend with a close girlfriend who was going through a rough time in her marriage, she invited her friend to lie down and practice yoga nidra meditation with her.

"We could have chosen to distract ourselves by going out to get food or doing something else together," Sarah told me, "but it didn't feel right to do that. It felt like we had to close the emotional loop, and respect it." Using yoga nidra helped them both be still and in the moment—together.

"It felt so beautiful to help hold this space for someone else, and of course myself," Sarah shared. "It felt wonderful to lie down with yoga nidra together and essentially say, let's feel."

Another beautiful way to share yoga nidra is with someone you are in conflict with. If you feel unable to forgive someone, perhaps practice yoga nidra a few times by yourself, but imagine the other person there, sharing in the peace and tranquility of yoga nidra with you. Then, if it feels right, invite that person to practice yoga nidra with you. This is a great first step to compassion and forgiveness when you don't have the words yet. But please invite others only when you feel well rested. I don't encourage women to share yoga nidra with anyone before they have nurtured themselves. This is a problem right now in our culture: we don't nurture ourselves. We help others feel better, we take care of them, from a state of exhaustion. And it's not working. This is why it's essential for you to experience the entire Daring to Rest program, let yourself be nurtured, and then share it when you're well rested. If you're a mom, I'm especially addressing you. Don't let the kids lie next to you while you practice yoga nidra unless you feel your cup is full. Give to yourself first, and then give to others from a well-rested place.

Yoga nidra is also a wonderful group activity for women who work together. I'm an activist and entrepreneur, and I work with many other women who are passionate about changing the world but wrestle with the passion that fuels their work. Burnout is well known to these women. But when they come together with other women to practice yoga nidra meditation, they begin to commit to their well-being on a deeper level. And then I get excited because this is the takeoff point to all transformation.

Remember: Chuck Perfect

Yoga nidra is now your friend for life. There will be days when you cannot practice yoga nidra meditation because you're needed elsewhere, and there will be days when life feels like it's falling apart. That's okay; yoga nidra is very forgiving. If you forget about it for a week, a month, or maybe even years, like I did, it will quickly welcome you back. All you do is lie back down and listen. And then listen to your soul whisper, a messenger that always knows: *You've got this.*

Optional: Practices to Stay Well-Rested for Life

Following are practices to help you embrace your well-rested woman. There's no perfect science to staying well rested, but it is essential that you develop ways to honestly check in with yourself and to use practices to stay connected to your most vital authentic self.

Assess How Rested You Are

Several years ago, I interviewed sleep specialist Dr. Rubin Naiman, and he pointed out that babies' lives revolve around three questions: (1) are they sleeping? (2) are they pooping? and (3) are they progressing developmentally? When we become adults, we stop asking these basic questions about our health and well-being. Yet he points out that when we don't ask them as adults we suffer, self-defeating habits continue, and exhaustion grows.

In the context of rest, these useful questions relate well to the three phases of the Daring to Rest program. Following is a Daring to Rest assessment to help you determine what phase needs your attention to help you feel healthy and well rested.

1. **Rest:** Am I rested in my body? Am I getting enough sleep? If you answered no to these questions, then your physical and energy bodies need attention. In addition to practicing the Phase One: Rest Meditation, use some of the optional practices to help balance these two bodies.

2. **Release:** Am I feeling peace and clarity of mind? Am I able to forgive others? Am I able to receive love from others? Is there something I'm not letting go of—anger, fear, or shame? Do I feel my wild nature? This is a phase where many people feel stuck. If this is you, give some attention to your mental, wisdom, and bliss bodies. Practice the Phase Two: Release Meditation and use some optional practices in chapters seven, eight, and nine to help balance these bodies.

3. **Rise:** Am I living my purpose? Am I following my big dreams from my heart? Do my dreams and purpose feel like an expression of my true nature? If you're holding back on living with purpose, or following a model of leading that feels too fast and out of sync with who you are, then it's time to pay attention to themes and do some of the optional practices in chapters ten and eleven. Lie down and practice the Phase Three: Rise Meditation.

Use Your Touchstone

Throughout the Daring to Rest journey, optional practices have invited you to use your touchstone on various parts of your body during your yoga nidra meditation. Now that your forty-day journey is coming to a close, here is one more way to keep using your touchstone.

Hold your touchstone in your hand with your eyes closed, ideally at your altar if you have created one. Imagine the insights you've had on your Daring to Rest journey, the first intention you started with, your soul whispers, and all your big dreams. Infuse your touchstone with the wisdom you've received during these forty days, welcoming both the dark and the light. Envision your well-rested woman, and if you wish, give your touchstone a name. Carry it with you or keep it on your altar or in your rest cave to remind you of your well-rested woman. Many pregnant women take their touchstone into their birth experience, menstruating women take it out during their periods, and menopausal women take it out when they feel hot flashes or any transitional moments. Another great time to keep it with you is monthly, on the full or new moon.

Refresh Your Altar or Rest Cave

If you created an altar and/or rest cave during your Daring to Rest journey, this is a great time to clean them up or change them up. Buy a new candle. Write down your current big dream or primary intention and place it in your space if you haven't already. Burn dried sage, cedar, or *palo santo* and wave it around your altar space. This clears old energy, so you can welcome your new, well-rested energy. Add items that invite vitality and align with your true nature, from poems to physical objects. You may want to place the soul whispers board or book that you created in chapter ten on your altar or in your cave and continue to add your new soul whispers. This is a great place to keep your essential oils if you're using them during your yoga nidra meditations.

Also, if you don't have time to communicate with your Council of Women during or just after your yoga nidra meditations, your altar or rest cave is a great place to come, light a candle, take a few slow, deep breaths, and ask them for guidance.

Optional: Diving Deeper

Looking to dive more deeply into your Daring to Rest journey and your future practice of yoga nidra? Consider these Daring to Rest optional prompts:

- What are three things you learned about yourself during your Daring to Rest journey? Freewrite about this topic.

- Freewrite in your journal about your soul whispers.

- Draw a picture of yourself living a well-rested lifestyle.

- Pick a song and dance to it as a well-rested woman. Consider using the song you heard in chapter ten as your "gold."

- What is your plan to practice yoga nidra moving forward? How often will you practice?

- List three people you want to share yoga nidra with and why. Describe how you would share yoga nidra with them. Be specific. (Where and when?)

Key Points in Chapter Eleven

- When crafting a well-rested lifestyle, it's important to see how all three phases of the Daring to Rest program—resting, releasing, and rising—are essential ingredients of the pie that is your life.

- To determine how much yoga nidra meditation you need after the Daring to Rest program, take the Daring to Rest assessment.

- Share yoga nidra meditation with others.

- Remember: *You've got this.*

Epilogue

FINAL YOGA NIDRA POMPOM SHAKE

Toward the end of writing this book, I bruised my left ribs badly when I slammed into a woman who set a blind pick during a game of three-on-three basketball. That evening, though it was clear why my ribs hurt, my body felt as though it were in mild shock. My mind was in overdrive, and sleeping, even breathing, was not going to be easy. So I put in my earbuds and plugged into a yoga nidra meditation. Not surprisingly, my body immediately calmed down.

The next morning, my husband took me to get an X-ray. Just getting out of bed was tough, and by the time we got to the radiology center, I was exhausted from the pain. After we checked in, I sat in the waiting room and plugged back into my yoga nidra meditation. As I was escorted to get X-rays, I felt deeply relaxed.

"How are you doing?" the technician asked as he adjusted my body in front of the machines.

"There is pain," I said, "but I've just been doing yoga nidra meditation, so I'm relaxed."

"I meditate," he said, "but I never heard of yoga nidra meditation."

By the end of the X-rays, I had told him all about yoga nidra: nap, meditation, deep sleep.

"You had me at *nap*," he said.

I smiled.

Back in the waiting room, my husband asked, "Why are you smiling?"

"Because he wants what I got," I said, remembering years ago when I had the same reaction the first time I found out there was a technique that combined meditation and sleep. I felt like I'd hit the meditation jackpot. I still do, which is why I keep shaking my yoga nidra pom-poms. And I hope now that you've discovered how well rested, peaceful, and alive you can feel with yoga nidra, you do too.

Welcome to the Daring to Rest sisterhood. It has been my pleasure to help you lie down to wake up. Keep daring to rest, chucking perfect, and dreaming big. You are enough.

Be good to yourself.

GRATITUDE

I am deeply thankful to all the women in my yoga nidra programs for your courage to rest. Your love and yoga nidra pompom-shaking with me have meant everything and have deeply informed this book.

A huge bow of gratitude to the women who shared their yoga nidra meditation stories with me for this book: Deborah, Mae, Monique, Margreet, Aditi, Tanya, Sarah, Maude, Cindy, Maria, Liz, Rachel, Genevieve, Billie, Charlene, and Judith. Some stories made it into the book, and many didn't, but all of your stories helped to elevate this book. Your enthusiasm for the magic of yoga nidra and the Daring to Rest program warms my heart.

To my editor, Amy Rost: I could not have written this book without you. The fact that you also have a great sense of humor and grace was beautiful icing on the cake.

Thanks to everyone on my team at Sounds True: especially Lindsey, Christine, and Sarah. You rock, women. And Jennifer Brown, thanks for believing in this book and for your positive, joyful nature.

To my agents, Janet Rosen and Sheree Bykofsky: Thanks for your faith in this book from the beginning.

To my yoga nidra mentors Kamini Desai, John Vosler, Renu, Yogi Amrit Desai, Anne Douglas, Robin Carnes, and Richard Miller: Your love for yoga nidra has touched me so very deeply and inspired me to share it with others.

To David Wright, for sharing your "Feminine Highway" exercise and all our incredible healing sessions. Thanks, my friend.

To the women in my writing and meditation group, Mary Hartley, Mert, Minal, Archie, Denise, Desiree, and Lezlie: Thanks for listening to very early drafts of this book and cheering me on as I wrote. Your sisterhood was invaluable.

To yogini and mamapreneur Alston Taggart, who believed in elevating yoga nidra to the next level, and in my vision, and spent hours helping me create all the initial design work. Your faith and friendship kept me dreaming big.

To Deborah Sullivan, thank you for providing the beautiful anointing rituals for the Rest, Release, and Rise phases. Your passionate love of yoga nidra, women, and the world inspires me. I have learned so much from you.

To Dr. Rubin Naiman, a sleep specialist who speaks the language of sleep medicine that our world so desperately needs to hear. When I found your book, everything I'd been observing about women's sleep issues made sense.

To Dr. Christiane Northrup, for courageously modeling how to change a women's health paradigm when I was a young woman looking for someone to boldly point out the obvious. And to all the new-paradigm health-care professionals who prescribe meditation and deep rest before medication.

To R.: Thank you for being my beautiful friend, inside and out, and for your poetic and often hilarious words that have lifted me to the highest vibration even at the lowest times. I love you.

To my father: You're always with me. Thanks for standing beside me, like a soul whisper, as I wrote this book.

To my mother: Thanks for your constant and unconditional support, love, and laughter. I feel so lucky every day.

To Tim, Jacob, and Aden: I now know why authors thank their families for all the sacrifices made to help their books get written. You guys made them all. Thanks for your love—always. I love you back. Your support helps me be bold in the world.

Finally, I thank Charlotte Perkins Gilman for daring *not* to rest. May it inspire women today to take back rest as a form of liberation.

Appendix 1

SCRIPTS FOR DARING TO REST YOGA NIDRA MEDITATIONS

You can download recordings of each of my yoga nidra meditations from the *Daring to Rest* page on the Sounds True website: SoundsTrue.com/daringtorest/yoganidrameditations. Or you can use the following scripts to record them in your own voice. They are best read slowly, clearly, and with frequent pauses. Also, keep your voice monotone—this isn't a theatrical reading. During the meditation, you do not want to be influenced by the emotional tone of any words.

Have a clock or watch with a second hand available so that you can time the specific pauses asked for in the scripts.

Phase One: Rest Meditation

Time: Approximately 15 minutes

Close your eyes.

Begin to feel yourself moving back from your everyday life. You're taking a journey to be good to yourself, to return to yourself, to rest deeply.

You're safe and protected in this space.

Water returns to a river, just as you return to yourself. Feel this.

(Pause for 10 seconds.)

Allow your body to be as comfortable as possible. Sink deep into the earth. Let the ground hold you. Relax. Let go.

Take a deep breath in, and exhale slowly, letting tension melt away.

Be still.

(Pause for 5 seconds.)

✳

Whether you consciously hear this voice guiding you or not,
there is a part of you that is always awake and will hear this voice.
You do not have to do anything.

You are now entering the yoga nidra cave. It's time to dare to rest and go within.

In this peaceful place, start feeling your Daring to Rest intention.

Repeat your intention to yourself. State it in the present tense—like, "I am a well-rested woman" or "I am whole"—as though it's happening right now.

Let your intention come from your heart, not your head. Feel it in your entire body.

(Pause for 10 seconds.)

✳

Now it's time to journey into the body. As a body part is named, feel any blocked energy dissolve, and allow that body part to relax deeply. *(Read the following list in the numbered order, but do not speak the numbers.)*

1. Space between the eyebrows

2. Hollow of the throat

3. Right shoulder joint

4. Right elbow joint

5. The bend of the right wrist joint

6. Tip of the right thumb

7. Tip of the right index finger

8. Tip of the right middle finger

9. Tip of the right fourth finger

10. Tip of the right small finger

11. The bend of the right wrist joint

12. Right elbow joint

13. Right shoulder joint

14. Hollow of the throat

15. Left shoulder joint

16. Left elbow joint

17. The bend of the left wrist joint

18. Tip of the left thumb

19. Tip of the left index finger

20. Tip of the left middle finger

21. Tip of the left fourth finger

22. Tip of the left small finger

23. The bend of the left wrist joint

24. Left elbow joint

25. Left shoulder joint

26. Hollow of the throat

27. Heart center

28. Right nipple

29. Heart center

30. Left nipple

31. Heart center

32. Solar plexus

33. Navel center

34. Right hip joint

35. Right knee joint

36. Right ankle joint

37. Tip of the right big toe

38. Tip of the right second toe

39. Tip of the right third toe

40. Tip of the right fourth toe

41. Tip of the right small toe

42. Right ankle joint

43. Right knee joint

44. Right hip joint

45. Navel center

46. Left hip joint

47. Left knee joint

48. Left ankle joint

49. Tip of the left big toe

50. Tip of the left second toe

51. Tip of the left third toe

52. Tip of the left fourth toe

53. Tip of the left small toe

54. Left ankle joint

55. Left knee joint

56. Left hip joint

57. Navel center

58. Solar plexus

59. Heart center

60. Hollow of the throat

61. Space between the eyebrows

Pay attention to all sensations in your body. Rest your mind.

If you have thoughts, picture yourself as a boat and the thoughts as extra things inside your hull. Slowly allow each thought to move over the side of the boat and into the water, where it gently floats away.

Soon you are an empty boat. Feel this sense of emptiness.

(Pause for 10 seconds.)

*

Notice your body breathing, the soft, gentle movement of the belly rising and falling. Inhale slowly, and exhale even more slowly. In and out. Releasing any worries and fears as you exhale. Noticing sensation in your body. Your body relaxing deeper. Welcome whatever you're feeling.

Now inhale slowly, filling the abdomen, then the chest, and all the way up to the neck. Exhale even more slowly, pursing your lips as if you're blowing through a straw.

And again—inhaling up to the neck, and exhaling like you're blowing through a straw.

Continue breathing like this for three more breaths.

(Pause for 10 seconds.)

Now stop, and notice sensations in your body. No judging, just welcoming everything. Noticing rhythm in your body, which areas feel in rhythm and which don't. Be present to all the energy in your body—and relax deeply into this vibration of energy.

(Pause for 10 seconds.)

*

Imagine yourself lying down on a red carpet in an open area of the woods. The sun is shining, majestic green trees surround you, and beside you is a beautiful waterfall. You hear the sound of the waterfall, and you feel the warmth of the sun on your entire body.

Slowly bring your awareness to the first power center, located between the tip of the tailbone and the bottom of the pubic bone.

Visualize bright red light moving through this area at the base of your spine. Notice any sensations here as you take a few slow, deep breaths in and out.

(Pause for 5 seconds.)

As you're lying on the carpet, deeply relaxed and warm, grounded to the earth, you notice the carpet's color turning to a deep, rich orange. You bring your awareness to the second power center, visualizing a deep orange color moving through your lower abdomen and into your reproductive area, lower back, and sacrum. Follow it with slow inhalations and exhalations.

Keep breathing.

Feel sensation. No thinking.

Listen to the sound of the waterfall as the orange begins to sink deeper and deeper into your lower spine and into your second power center. Relax and feel.

(Pause for 10 seconds.)

Now bring your attention to the space between your eyebrows and rest here. Let go of all fears. Experience total peace and stillness.

Witness a light inside of you come on, your internal power switch.

Feel this.

Be this.

Relax in total peace and tranquility.

(Pause for 30 seconds.)

*

Repeat your intention three times.

(Pause for 10 seconds.)

Say hello to it—"I see you." And then let it be planted like a seed into the depths of the rich, moist soil.

❋

Now repeat the following affirmations. Absorb each affirmation as if you're digesting it into your entire system. Feel it permeate every cell and atom. *(Pause for 5 seconds between each affirmation.)*

- I am grounded, safe, and supported.

- My life force is flowing freely, opening all channels for healing.

- I am filled with creative energy and vitality.

Notice your connection to the earth, your heart beating, life force flowing, in you and outside of you, to infinity.

(Pause for 5 seconds.)

Notice sensation in front of the body, behind the body, to the left of the body, to the right, above, and below the body.

If there's any area of your body that needs healing, send light to that area now.

(Pause for 10 to 15 seconds.)

❋

Now take a deep breath in through your heart. Follow your breath and see where it lands in your body.

Wherever the breath arrives, notice if there's an image, word, or phrase that's being whispered to you. No thinking, just feel this whisper.

This is your soul whisper.

Be grateful for whatever you received.

And now be still and notice the impact of your soul whisper in the form of sensations on your body and in your mind.

(Pause for 10 seconds.)

Everything is okay.

Feel this.

Notice how peaceful your body feels. Come out of your body for a moment and observe yourself experiencing deep peace and relaxation. Vow to take this peace back into your everyday life, or if you plan to go to sleep now, take this peace into your sleep.

Repeat your intention again three times.

(Pause for 10 seconds.)

Trust that it has been heard and will act as a compass back to your power.

* * *

Now, feeling deeply relaxed, begin to emerge from your yoga nidra nap.

Notice the sweet sensation of rest in your body. Carry it into your day, your sleep, your life.

Spend a little more time sending love to any area of your body that needs it today.

(Pause for 10 seconds.)

Now, if you're getting up, open your eyes slowly.

And with micro-movements, begin to move your body, starting anywhere that feels right to you. Let your body decide when and how it will move.

Your breath is soft; your mind is clear.

Yoga nidra is complete.

Be good to yourself.

Phase Two: Release Meditation

Time: Approximately 30 minutes

Close your eyes.

Now begin to imagine you're lying or sitting in a warm, cozy cave, in a zone of total silence.

If you hear noise, let it invite you to go deeper into your cave.

Feel yourself in the cave, sensing your body, and connecting deeply to the earth—tapping into fluidity, ease, and stillness.

Notice all the elements:

- The ground beneath you—earth

- A trickle of rain outside the cave—water

- The fresh smell of the cave meeting your skin—air

- And the warmth of the cave—fire

Be still.

"Release . . . release . . . release," you whisper to yourself.

Trust in the profound pauses. You cannot have rest unless you pause.

Feel yourself moving into the pause, whatever this means to you.

(Pause for 5 seconds.)

Take a deep breath in, and stretch your mouth open as wide as you can. Hold your mouth stretched open for a count of three.

Hold . . .

Hold . . .

Hold . . .

Now release with a sigh, letting go of any holding in the body.

(Pause for 5 seconds.)

And again, take a deep breath in and open your mouth wide, stretching it as wide as you can.

Hold . . .

Hold . . .

Hold . . .

Now release.

Relax. Be still.

(Pause for 5 seconds.)

*

It's time to turn on your internal power switch.

Take a moment to notice vibration in your body—your life force.

Now shift gears from doing mode to doing absolutely nothing. Just be.

(Pause for 5 seconds.)

Do nothing from now on except follow the voice. Stay awake and alert. If you fall asleep, you will still benefit from yoga nidra, but try to stay awake until the end. You cannot do yoga nidra wrong, so give up perfection and just listen and relax.

Permission to rest is granted. You are entering the yoga nidra cave. It's time to dare to rest and go within.

(Pause for 5 seconds.)

*

Repeat your intention to yourself three times. If there is a specific intention you wish to plant, to help you release a habit or pattern, make your intention a positive statement of the heartfelt intention you wish to grow. Be sure your intention is stated in the present tense, like it's happening right now.

(Pause for 10 seconds.)

Let all sensations associated with your intention spread throughout your body.

*

Now we'll rotate attention through the feminine landscape of your body. Do not visualize the body part, but instead notice sensation when the body part is mentioned. If you have had that body part removed, there is still energy associated with that area, so tune into the energy in that area of the body.

Begin with noticing sensation in
the space between your eyebrows,
mouth,
nose,

left eye,
right eye,
both eyes,
left ear,
right ear,
both ears,
forehead,
back of the head,
back of the neck,
throat,
right shoulder,
left shoulder,
both shoulders,
right arm,
left arm,
both arms,
right hand,
left hand,
both hands,
throat,
middle of the chest,
right breast,
left breast,
both breasts,
navel point,
right ovary,
left ovary,
both ovaries,
uterus,
cervix,
right fallopian tube,
left fallopian tube,
both fallopian tubes,
vagina,
pubic bone,

right hip,
left hip,
both hips,
right leg,
left leg,
both legs,
right foot,
left foot,
both feet,
back of the legs,
lower back,
middle back,
upper back,
back of the neck,
throat,
and back to the space between your eyebrows.
Rest in this space. Observe stillness.

(Pause for 15 seconds.)

*

Begin to notice the breath moving through the space between your eyebrows.

As you breathe in, the belly rises, entering the space between the eyebrows.

And as you breathe out, the belly falls, and the breath exits your body through the space between the eyebrows, allowing any stagnation in the body to leave.

Breathe in and out from this spot at your own pace.

Follow the breath. Let it decide the pace.

(Pause for 10 seconds.)

✳

Now, from the space between your eyebrows, inhale slowly down to the base of your spine while saying the sound *Soooooo* to yourself.

Then slowly exhale from the base of the spine back up to the space between your eyebrows while silently saying the sound *Hummmmmm.*

Feel your awareness expanding and merging with your life force.

Continue breathing and repeating the *So Hum* chant silently in rhythm with your breath.

Breathing in *Soooooo* from the space between your eyebrows to the base of the spine.

And exhaling *Hummmmmm,* the breath moving from the base of the spine back to the space between your eyebrows.

(Pause for 10 seconds.)

Now remain in your third eye and feel all sensation in your body. Welcome everything.

(Pause for 5 seconds.)

✳

Remember an experience you have had of feeling disconnected, weak, powerless. Feel this in your body, but do not concentrate on its source. Feel the experience of feeling powerless as clearly as possible.

(Pause for 10 seconds.)

Now allow the opposite feeling to rise—feeling powerful, connected, in the body and your entire mind. You are feeling powerful.

(Pause for 10 seconds.)

Now welcome both feelings. Breathe in and out as you feel both powerless and powerful.

(Pause for 10 seconds.)

*

Remember an experience you have had of feeling confusion and numbness. Feel this in your body, but do not concentrate on its source. Re-create the experience of feeling confused and numb as clearly as possible.

(Pause for 5 seconds.)

Now allow the opposite feeling to rise, feeling clarity and luminousness in the body and your entire mind. You are feeling clear and open, intuitive.

(Pause for 5 seconds.)

Now welcome both feelings. Breathe in and out as you feel both confusion and clarity.

(Pause for 10 seconds.)

*

Begin to visualize yourself walking on a beach, your feet kissing the sand. You are breathing in and out slowly as you walk.

There's a bonfire ahead of you, and you walk toward it.

When you arrive at the bonfire, there's a warm glow from the flames. Feel this warmth in your cells.

(Pause for 10 seconds.)

Now lie down on the sand. You're deeply relaxed, the sand against your back. Total connection to the earth. The sound of the ocean—water. Your skin notices the fresh ocean breeze—air. And you feel the bonfire in every atom and cell of your being.

Open your senses to all of this. Feel how your body aligns with the frequency of earth, water, air, and fire.

Now, from this place of total relaxation and deep connection, where do you feel a yes in your body?

(Pause for 5 seconds.)

Where do you feel a no?

(Pause for 5 seconds.)

Now how does it feel to feel both yes and no? Just notice. Be kind and gentle with whatever is rising as you hold both yes and no. You don't need to put a story to it, just see how you feel.

(Pause for 10 seconds.)

As you're lying down, notice a yellow, sparkling light at your abdomen—your gut. Let your entire digestive area fill with this yellow sparkle.

Imagine a bridge between your body and your soul. Begin to move from body into soul and notice how this feels. What does soul feel like to you?

Just notice. Let go of your thinking mind. Pay attention to sensation only.

(Pause for 5 seconds.)

As you're lying down in your soul, connected to your life force, opening to wisdom, notice an indigo sparkle in the space between your eyebrows.

The sparkle moves up to the crown of your head, turning white. Allow this white light to activate your internal power switch, sending healing to dissolve all shame, any parts of your body that have been betrayed, and all feelings of not being enough.

(Pause for 5 seconds.)

Welcome a new relationship with yourself as a woman.

(Pause for 10 seconds.)

Now, from your position next to the fire, look up at the sky and see if there's a healing message for you in the stars.

(Pause for 10 seconds.)

You feel a glow in your heart, and you know everything is okay.

You are okay.

Feel this.

Be true to your feelings, whatever they are. Welcome them as you sit, completely empty of all thoughts, connected to your internal power switch.

(Pause for 10 seconds.)

Watch the fire, and slowly begin to imagine an emotion or habit or pattern that you are ready to release. It could be anger or fear. Or maybe it's a behavior you want to release.

Feel this piece of emotional exhaustion in your body. Bless it, and then release it into the fire. Let it go.

Now watch what you've released burn as if you're witnessing it like a movie. Notice all the sensations in your body as you watch it burning in the fire.

(Pause for 10 seconds.)

*

Bring your attention to the space between your eyebrows. Remain deeply relaxed. Your breath is soft and at ease.

You're in a safe container of tranquility, love, and deep silence. Feel and experience this.

You are free.

It's here your Wild Woman emerges.

Feel her presence within you.

Completely let go of fear and anxiety.

Relax. Be wild. Be calm. Be free.

Feel this.

(Pause for 30 seconds.)

*

Repeat your intention three times.

(Pause for 10 seconds.)

Let it go to the deepest levels of your being. Trust that whether you know it or not, every cell, every atom, every part of you hears your intention and invites it to come toward you.

(Pause for 5 seconds.)

*

Now affirm the following statements. Listen deeply, and feel each statement in your body. Let the feeling come from your heart. *(Pause for 5 seconds after each statement.)*

- I am a free-flowing river—connected, powerful, and robust.

- I release what does not serve me and realize my full potential.

- I am connected to my inner knowing at all times.

- I hear my Wild Woman, and my heart is always open to receiving her.

*

Now notice a circle of women surrounding you.

This is your Council of Women. They can be women you know or women you don't know. They can be living or have passed on. They are mentors, guides, seers.

Welcome whomever arrives. Receive their love and sisterhood.

(Pause for 5 seconds.)

Know you are never alone. You are supported and connected to their love.

If you have a question that you need guidance on, ask them now.

(Pause for 15 seconds.)

As they leave, fill your heart with a smile. Notice how this feels.

(Pause for 5 seconds.)

❉

Take a deep breath in through your heart. Follow your breath and see where it lands in your body.

Wherever the breath arrives, see if there's an image, word, or phrase that's being whispered to you. This is your soul whisper.

(Pause for 10 seconds.)

Whatever you receive, be curious and openhearted. Vow to honor your soul whisper.

See it.

Listen deeply.

Now notice how you feel.

(Pause for 10 seconds.)

*

Repeat your intention again three times.

(Pause for 5 seconds.)

Imagine your intention happening. Allow it to spread throughout your body and then to all the open space around you—and to infinity.

*

Ever so slowly, begin the process of waking up, first noticing what body part wishes to move first and then beginning to move from this place.

Tiny movements.

Staying safe and cozy and relaxed.

Moving at your own pace, when it feels right.

And as you're moving, being aware of your body, back and front of the body, right and left sides, above and below—your whole body.

And beyond your body. How far beyond your body can you feel into?

You're slowly transitioning out of yoga nidra. The breath is slow and peaceful. Your mind is relaxed. It's quiet.

Take a few more moments to notice how it feels in your body to be quiet.

(Pause for 5 seconds.)

Now, if it feels right, bend your knees and bring them to your chest. Rock side to side, eventually moving to your right side, curled in a fetal position, arms crossed like you're hugging yourself. Or if you're sitting, you're bending forward, your arms hugging yourself.

Be aware of how deeply you now know yourself again—your true authentic self—the Wild Woman—the woman with her internal power switch on—the woman who knows she's worthy and enough—and who chucks perfect, always.

If you're waking up, start to sit up, open your eyes. If you're continuing on to sleep, enjoy sweet, cozy dreams.

This completes yoga nidra.

Be good to yourself.

Phase Three: Rise Meditation

Time: Approximately 40 minutes

Close your eyes and begin to quiet your mind—for peace of mind.

It's time to transition from busyness to ease, from time-bound to timeless.

(Pause for 5 seconds.)

This is your time to dare to rest.

Allow yourself to begin to relax.

Become aware of all sounds. Start with distant sounds. No straining—just notice the sounds you hear outside.

Then begin to pull back, toward the room you're in, and listen for sounds closer to you. Keep drawing your attention inward, aware of sounds, until you're inside your body.

Notice any sounds inside your body.

Be still.

(Pause for 5 to 10 seconds.)

*

From here, visualize the space you're in. See yourself lying down or sitting in this space, practicing yoga nidra.

The position of your body . . . the expression on your face . . . your clothes . . . your hair. Like a movie . . . visualize yourself practicing yoga nidra.

Take a deep breath in. And exhale, releasing tension all over your body.

(Pause for 5 seconds.)

And now take another deep breath. Breathing in. And out, releasing stress and worry.

(Pause for 5 seconds.)

Let go. Let the ground or the chair hold you.

Allow your inhalations and exhalations to become longer and slower, without effort, moving into a slow, rhythmic breath.

(Pause for 5 seconds.)

*

During yoga nidra, stay awake and alert. Follow the guidance of this voice at all times.

Remain relaxed.

There's nothing to do, nowhere to be.

Permission to rest is now granted.

You're entering the yoga nidra cave. It's time to dare to rest and go within.

*

Now repeat your intention with your full awareness three times, feeling it in every part of your body. It should be short, in simple language that's true to you, and in the present tense.

Maybe your intention is a big dream, maybe not. Whatever it is, open to it.

Spend a few moments feeling your intention.

(Pause for 5 seconds.)

*

Now begin by bringing your awareness to
the right-hand thumb,
index finger,
middle finger,
ring finger,
little finger,
palm of the hand,
back of the hand,
wrist,
forearm,
elbow,
upper arm,
shoulder,
armpit,
pubic bone,
right hip,
thigh,
knee,
calf,
ankle,
heel,
sole of the right foot,
top of the foot,
right big toe,
second toe,
third toe,

fourth toe,
and fifth toe.
Now moving to the left side of the body, starting with
the left-hand thumb,
index finger,
middle finger,
ring finger,
little finger,
palm of the hand,
back of the hand,
wrist,
forearm,
elbow,
upper arm,
shoulder,
armpit,
pubic bone,
left hip,
thigh,
knee,
calf,
ankle,
heel,
sole of the left foot,
top of the foot,
left big toe,
second toe,
third toe,
fourth toe,
and fifth toe.
Now bringing your awareness to the back of the body,
right heel,
left heel,
right calf,
left calf,

right thigh,
left thigh,
right buttock,
left buttock,
lower back,
middle back,
upper back,
the whole spine,
right shoulder blade,
left shoulder blade,
back of the neck,
back of the head,
top of the head,
forehead,
right temple,
left temple,
right ear,
left ear,
right eyebrow,
left eyebrow,
space between the eyebrows,
right eye,
left eye,
right nostril,
left nostril,
right cheek,
left cheek,
upper lip,
lower lip,
the space where both lips meet,
chin,
jaw,
throat,
right collarbone,
left collarbone,

right side of the chest,
left side of the chest,
right breast,
left breast,
middle of the chest,
upper abdomen,
navel,
lower abdomen,
right ovary,
left ovary,
uterus,
cervix,
vagina,
the entire pelvic floor,
the whole right leg,
whole left leg,
whole right arm,
whole left arm,
the whole face,
whole head,
whole torso,
and the whole body.
Become aware of your whole body.
Bathe in sensation.
Feel your whole body.

(Pause for 5 seconds.)

Rest here. Notice sensations that arise.

What are you gestating?

A creative project?

A baby?

A business?

Surround what you are gestating in light, keeping it as sacred in your womb.

Breathe in slowly, and as you breathe out, release anything you need to clear your womb space so that you may welcome what you're gestating even more, so you may rise up to this new birth.

Feel this.

(Pause for 5 seconds.)

*

And now bring your awareness to the space between your eyebrows.

(Pause for 10 seconds.)

Breath and body, one movement.

Breathe in and out on the left side of your body three times.

(Pause for 5 seconds.)

Now breathe in and out on the right side three times.

(Pause for 5 seconds.)

Breathe in and out in front of your body three times.

(Pause for 5 seconds.)

Breathe in and out in back of your body three times. Feel all boundaries of the body dissolving.

(Pause for 15 seconds.)

*

Bring your awareness to the base of your spine. Breathe in and out the color red from the base of your spine.

Slow inhalations and even slower exhalations.

Breathing in and out red from the base of your spine.

(Pause for 10 seconds.)

Now move to your sacral area, and breathe in and out a deep orange color from the sacrum.

In, and out, slowly.

(Pause for 10 seconds.)

Moving up to your digestive area, your abdomen, breathing in and out the color yellow.

Breathing slowly, steady, in . . . and out.

(Pause for 10 seconds.)

Now breathing from your heart the color green, in and out, slowly.

Allow the breath to be rhythmic, a beautiful green color flowing in and out from your heart.

(Pause for 10 seconds.)

On your next inhalation, move into your throat, and begin to breathe in and out a vibrant blue.

In . . . and out.

Noticing sensation as you breathe.

(Pause for 10 seconds.)

Now moving to the space between your eyebrows, begin to breathe in and out a deep, dark blue-violet, indigo, from this space.

Breathing in indigo and out indigo.

Notice the flow in and out.

Relax.

(Pause for 10 seconds.)

On the next inhalation, move up to the top of your head, and here breathe in white light for several breaths.

(Pause for 10 seconds.)

Now begin to breathe the white light through your entire body.

A healing white light, moving into all parts of your body.

Your body filling with white light.

(Pause for 10 seconds.)

Notice sensation in your body. Your senses are wide open.

(Pause for 10 seconds.)

*

Start counting backward from twenty-one to one, like this:

Twenty-one, I am breathing in.

Twenty-one, I am breathing out.

Twenty, I am breathing in.

Twenty, I am breathing out.

Continue at your own pace, from twenty-one to one. If you lose count, return to the beginning.

(Pause for 30 seconds.)

Breathing slowly, counting down to one.

(Pause for 20 seconds.)

Counting and breathing.

(Pause for 10 seconds.)

Stop counting. Notice sensation in your body.

(Pause for 15 seconds.)

*

Begin to feel your body is light as air.
Your head, light as a feather.
Neck, light as a feather.
Shoulders, light.

Arms, light and relaxed.
Chest and abdomen, light.
Your ovaries, light as a feather.
Uterus, light. Your hips, light and airy.
Both legs and feet, light.
Your whole body, light, like it's floating.
Feel this.

(Pause for 15 seconds.)

And now bring a sensation of heaviness to your body. Your body feels heavy, as if it's sinking into the floor.

Each body part heavy, from head to toes.

Bring heaviness to your whole body.

Immerse yourself in feeling heavy.

(Pause for 15 seconds.)

And now feel both light and heavy.

How does it feel to feel both at the same time?

Just notice. Don't think your way—feel your way.

What sensations are you feeling when you hold both?

(Pause for 15 seconds.)

*

Notice how the following statements feel in your body. Be sure to not think your way, but instead feel your way:

"I am unworthy."

Feel this. If you need to, bring up a memory. And then drop the memory and stay with the feeling.

(Pause for 15 seconds.)

"I am worthy."

Feel this. If you need to, bring up a memory. And then drop the memory and stay with the feeling.

(Pause for 15 seconds.)

"I am not enough."

Feel this. If you need to, bring up a memory. And then drop the memory and stay with the feeling.

(Pause for 15 seconds.)

"I am enough."

Feel this. If you need to, bring up a memory. And then drop the memory and stay with the feeling.

(Pause for 15 seconds.)

"I strive for perfection."

Feel this. If you need to, bring up a memory. And then drop the memory and stay with the feeling.

(Pause for 15 seconds.)

"I let go of perfection."

Feel this. If you need to, bring up a memory. And then drop the memory and stay with the feeling.

(Pause for 15 seconds.)

"I feel shame."

Feel this. If you need to, bring up a memory. And then drop the memory and stay with the feeling.

(Pause for 15 seconds.)

"I feel no shame."

Feel this. If you need to, bring up a memory. And then drop the memory and stay with the feeling.

(Pause for 15 seconds.)

*

In this state of deep relaxation, begin to visualize yourself in a golden temple, a sacred space on a mountaintop.

You're lying down, in a deep state of peace and tranquility. No fear, no anxiety, completely at rest.

If there are any areas of tension in the body, release the tension now. Release until you feel completely at ease.

(Pause for 10 seconds.)

Your whole body is empty.

Now you get to decide what creative energy you want to bring into it. Bring your awareness to your womb. Allow this creative energy to start in the womb and then go to any area of the body that needs healing.

This energy may be something specific, like a creative idea, or not. It's creative energy you want to give your well-rested woman, to help her dream big.

Take a moment to let this creative energy make itself known as a color. Bathe your whole body and beyond your body, into infinity, in this color.

Don't think your way—feel.

(Pause for 15 seconds.)

Witness yourself with this new creative energy.

(Pause for 15 seconds.)

*

Now bring your attention to the space between your eyebrows and do absolutely nothing.

Be still.

Here you are turning on your internal power switch. Feel your Wild Woman arrive.

(Pause for 5 seconds.)

Now feel grace—be grace.

Relax and completely let go into the deepest peace.

(Pause for 30 seconds.)

*

From this peaceful place, bring your intention into your awareness.

Repeat your intention now three times to yourself. Feel it deep in your entire being, like an intravenous drip flowing into all parts of you.

(Pause for 10 seconds.)

*

Repeat the following affirmations. *(Pause for 5 seconds between each affirmation.)*

- I am a Wild Woman.

- I am well rested.

- I dream big from a well-rested place.

*

Now notice a circle of women surrounding you.

This is your Council of Women. They can be women you know or women you don't know. They can be living or have passed on. They are mentors, guides, seers.

Welcome them. Receive their love and sisterhood. And perhaps guidance, if you need it.

(Pause for 15 seconds.)

Know you are never alone. You are supported and connected to their love.

As they slowly leave, fill your heart with a smile.

*

Take a deep breath in through your heart. Follow your breath and see where it lands in your body.

Wherever the breath arrives, see if there's an image, word, or phrase that's being whispered to you. This is your soul whisper.

(Pause for 10 seconds.)

Whatever you receive, be curious and openhearted. Vow to honor your soul whisper.

See it.

Listen deeply.

Now notice how you feel.

(Pause for 10 seconds.)

*

Become aware of how relaxed the body feels. Take a few final moments to move through your seven power centers,

starting at the base of your spine, seeing a red sparkle of light, then moving to your sacrum, and a deep orange sparkle,

on to your abdomen, a yellow sparkle,

moving into the heart, seeing a green sparkle,

now the throat, and a blue sparkle,

moving into the space between the eyebrows, seeing an indigo sparkle,

and now at top of the head, seeing a white sparkle.

If there are any areas of the body that need healing, send white light to those areas now.

(Pause for 5 seconds.)

*

As you begin to transition out of yoga nidra, repeat your intention again to yourself.

(Pause for 5 seconds.)

Feel yourself shifting into alignment with your intention.

(Pause for 5 seconds.)

Do nothing. Trust in your intention—that it's just right and will serve you well.

*

Notice what part of your body has the desire to move. Follow this desire and move that body part.

Then notice what body part wants to move next, and move from that place. Micro-movements.

If you're drifting off to sleep, let your body adjust for sleep.

If you are waking up, open your eyes slowly. Begin to notice the room around you—sounds, smells, your breath, your body, your intuition, your worthiness, your enoughness.

Feel all of this inside of your body, outside of your body.

Feel down to Mother Earth and up to Father Sky. Unite the two. Feel them come together.

Feel your true nature. And know you are a well-rested woman.

Yoga nidra is complete.

Be good to yourself.

Appendix 2

YOUR DARING TO REST TOOLBOX

T he Daring to Rest program provides practice tools you can use forever. When you need to address physical exhaustion, you'll choose the rest tools. If you feel emotionally exhausted, you'll dive into the release tools. And for life-purpose exhaustion, you'll use the rise-up practices.

Let intuition tell you when and how to apply the tools. If one doesn't stand out as right for you, write the names of the tools on separate pieces of paper and place them face down. Mix them up. Then take three slow, deep breaths and, with your left hand, pick a piece of paper. This is the tool to use.

Following is a list of all the practices/tools mentioned throughout the book and the chapters they are in, so you can find them easily when you need them.

Phase One: Rest
The focus is addressing physical exhaustion.

Intention (Chapter Four)
- Discovering Your Intention

Body (Chapter Five)
- Activate the First Power Center
- Anointing Practice for the Rest Phase
- Lie on the Ground
- Sixty-One-Point Relaxation
- Mindful Movement
- Open Your Feminine Highway

Energy (Chapter Six)
- Activate the Second Power Center
- Use Water
- Cooling Breath
- Alternate Nostril Breathing
- Pay Attention to Rhythm

Phase Two: Release

The focus of this phase is releasing emotions, thoughts, and habits that no longer serve you and keep you from feeling peace of mind.

Mind (Chapter Seven)
- Holding Opposites Practice
- Activate Your Third Power Center
- Anointing Practice for the Release Phase
- Clean Out Your Gut
- The Ha Breath
- Create a New Intention

Wisdom (Chapter Eight)
- Connect to Your Council of Women
- Activate Your Soul
- *So Hum* Breath
- Tapping Your Thymus

Bliss (Chapter Nine)
- Activate Your Fourth Power Center
- Inhale Joy
- Laugh
- Nurture Others

Phase Three: Rise

This phase focuses on rising up in your life in a new way, so you can make a difference and continue to feel well rested.

Lead (Chapter Ten)
- Four Steps for Discovering Your Big Dreams
- Activate the Fifth and Sixth Power Centers
- Anointing Practice for the Rise Phase
- Practice Sensing and Saying Yes and No
- Love Yourself First (give kindness, go on wonder dates)

Life (Chapter Eleven)
- Assess How Rested You Are
- Use Your Touchstone
- Refresh Your Altar or Rest Cave

NOTES

Chapter 1   Why Rest Is So Important for Women

1. National Sleep Foundation, *2014 Sleep Health Index* (Arlington, VA: The National Sleep Foundation, 2014), sleepfoundation.org/sites/default/files/2014%20Sleep %20Health%20Index-FINAL_0.PDF.

2. D. J. Taylor et al., "Epidemiology of Insomnia, Depression, and Anxiety," *Sleep* 28, no. 11 (2005):1462.

3. Medco Health Solutions, "America's State of Mind: New Report Finds Americans Increasingly Turn to Medications to Ease Their Mental Woes; Women Lead the Trend," *PR Newswire*, November 16, 2011, prnewswire.com/news-releases /americas-state-of-mind-new-report-finds-americans-increasingly-turn-to-medications-to-ease-their-mental-woes-women-lead-the-trend-133939038.html.

4. L. A. Pratt, D. J. Brody, and Q. Gu, "Antidepressant Use in Persons Aged 12 and Over: United States, 2005–2008," *NCHS Data Brief* no. 76 (Hyattsville, MD: National Center for Health Statistics, 2011), 2, cdc.gov/nchs/data/databriefs /db76.pdf.

5. Rubin R. Naiman, *Healing Night: The Science and Spirit of Sleeping, Dreaming, and Awakening* (Minneapolis: Syren Book Company, 2006), 41.

6. David Whyte, "Rest," in *Consolations: The Solace, Nourishment and Underlying Meaning of Everyday Words* (Langley, WA: Many Rivers Press, 2016), 181.

7. Nathaniel Kleitman, *Sleep and Wakefulness*, rev. ed. (Chicago: University of Chicago Press, 1987).

8. Nathaniel Kleitman, "Basic Rest-Activity Cycle—22 Years Later," *Sleep* 5, no. 4 (December 1982): 311–17.

9. Naiman, *Healing Night*, 41.

10. DeLisa Fairweather, Sylvia Frisancho-Kiss, and Noel R. Rose, "Sex Differences in Autoimmune Disease from a Pathological Perspective," *The American Journal of Pathology* 173, no. 3 (September 2008): 600–609.

11. Clarissa Pinkola Estés, *Women Who Run With the Wolves: Myths and Stories of the Wild Woman Archetype* (New York: Ballantine, 1992), 427.

Chapter 2   Welcome to Yoga Nidra

1. Swami Satyananda Saraswati, *Yoga Nidra* (Munger, Bihar, India: Yoga Publications Trust, 1998), 14; Kamakhya Kumar, "Complete the Course of Sleep through Yoga Nidra," *Nature and Wealth* 7, no. 1 (January 2008): 8.

2. Khushbu Rani, S. Tiwari, U. Singh, et al., "Impact of Yoga Nidra on Psychological General Wellbeing in Patients with Menstrual Irregularities: A Randomized Controlled Trial," *International Journal of Yoga* 4, no. 1 (2011): 20.

3. Kamakhya Kumar, *A Handbook of Yoga Nidra* (New Delhi, India: D.K. Printworld, 2013), 56.

4. Pranav Pandya and Kamakhya Kumar, "Yoga Nidra and Its Impact on Human Physiology," *Yoga Vijnana* 1, no. 1 (2007): 1–8; S. Amita, S. Prabhakar, I. Manoj, et al., "Effect of Yoga-Nidra on Blood Glucose Level in Diabetic Patients," *Indian Journal of Physiology and Pharmacology* 53, no. 1 (January–March 2009): 97–101.

5. Pamela G. Pence, Lori S. Katz, Cristi Huffman, et al., "Delivering Integrative Restoration–Yoga Nidra Meditation (iRest) to Women with Sexual Trauma at a Veteran's Medical Center: A Pilot Study," *International Journal of Yoga Therapy*, no. 24 (2014), irest.us/sites/default/files/iRest%20for %20Women%20with%20Sexual%20Trauma%202014 _Research,Pence_0.pdf.
Also see Courtney Hartman, "Exploring the Experiences of Women with Complex Trauma with the Practice of iRest–Yoga

Nidra" (doctoral dissertation, California Institute of Integral Studies, 2015), irest.us/sites/default/files/iRest%20and %20Women%20with%20Complex%20Trauma.pdf.

6. Richard Miller, *The iRest Program for Healing PTSD: A Proven-Effective Approach to Using Yoga Nidra Meditation and Deep Relaxation Techniques to Overcome Trauma* (Oakland, CA: New Harbinger Publications, 2015).

Phase One   Rest

1. Naiman, *Healing Night*, 40.

Chapter 6   Energy

1. Marcus E. Raichle and Debra A. Gusnard, "Appraising the Brain's Energy Budget," *Proceedings of the National Academy of Sciences* 99, no. 16 (August 2002): 10, 237–39.

Phase Two   Release

1. Marianne Williamson, *Illuminata: A Return to Prayer* (New York: Riverhead Books, 1995), 149.

2. R. Stevens, "Working against Our Endogenous Circadian Clock: Breast Cancer and Electric Lighting in the Modern World," *Mutation Research* 680, nos.1–2 (November–December 2009): 106–8.

Chapter 7   Mind

1. Daniel Goleman, *Emotional Intelligence: Why It Can Matter More Than IQ* (New York: Bantam, 2006), 207.

2. Viktor E. Frankl, *Man's Search for Meaning* (1946; repr. Boston: Beacon Press, 2006), 66.

3. Michael J. Breus, "Unlocking the Sleep-Gut Connection," Huffington Post, January 13, 2016, huffingtonpost. com/dr-michael-j-breus/unlocking-the-sleep-gut-connection_b_8941314.html.

Chapter 8 Wisdom

1. Estés, *Women Who Run With the Wolves*, 22.
2. Ibid., 125.

Phase Three Rise

1. Charlotte Perkins Gilman, "Why I Wrote *The Yellow Wallpaper?*" *The Forerunner* (October 1913), nlm.nih.gov /exhibition/theliteratureofprescription/exhibitionAssets /digitalDocs/WhyIWroteYellowWallPaper.pdf.

Chapter 10 Lead

1. ALisa Starkweather, "I am sad tonight, and I don't think I'm alone," Facebook post, February 7, 2017, facebook.com/photo .php?fbid=10154922228026763&set=a.53616791762.79395. 672291762&type=3&theater.
2. Valerie Estelle Frankel, *From Girl to Goddess: The Heroine's Journey through Myth and Legend* (Jefferson, NC: McFarland, 2010), 20.

Chapter 11 Life

1. Marion Woodman, *Holding the Tension of the Opposites* (audiobook) (Boulder, CO: Sounds True, 1994), 1 cassette; 00:45.
2. Estés, *Women Who Run With the Wolves*, 20.

RECOMMENDED READING

Looking for books to read on your Daring to Rest journey? Here are some of my favorites.

Brogan, Kelly. *A Mind of Your Own: The Truth About Depression and How Women Can Heal Their Bodies to Reclaim Their Lives.* New York: Harper Wave, 2016. I started doing backflips when I read this bold book that essentially shows you why you're not crazy and how you can naturally heal.

Brown, Brené. *Daring Greatly: How the Courage to Be Vulnerable Transforms the Way We Live, Love, Parent, and Lead.* New York: Avery, 2012. Makes data on vulnerability feel sexy and inspiring.

Chödrön, Pema. *When Things Fall Apart: Heart Advice for Difficult Times.* Boulder, CO: Shambhala, 2002. Always on my bedside table.

Cohen, Doris. *Repetition: Past Lives, Life, and Rebirth.* Carlsbad, CA: Hay House, 2008. Fascinating read with practical advice you can follow at home. It's a great complement to the Release phase of the Daring to Rest program. I love this book, and women in my programs do too!

Desai, Kamini. *Yoga Nidra: The Art of Transformational Sleep.* New Delhi, India: Lotus Press, 2017. This yoga nidra book from my mentor is a comprehensive guidebook exploring yogic philosophy and modern-day yoga nidra.

Huffington, Arianna. *The Sleep Revolution: Transforming Your Life, One Night at a Time.* New York: Harmony, 2016. Simply the best one-stop shopping for information on sleep.

Kent, Tami Lynn. *Wild Feminine: Finding Power, Spirit, and Joy in the Core of the Female Body.* Hillsboro, OR: Beyond Words, 2011. This book will make you feel powerful and proud to be a woman.

Miller, Richard. *The iRest Program for Healing PTSD: A Proven-Effective Approach to Using Yoga Nidra Meditation and Deep Relaxation Techniques to Overcome Trauma.* Oakland, CA: New Harbinger Publications, 2015. Learn about iRest yoga nidra's unique and successful approach to healing PTSD.

Mohr, Tara. *Playing Big: Find Your Voice, Your Mission, Your Message.* Nottingham, UK: Hutchinson, 2014. Full of practical advice on how women can lead with heart and soul.

Naiman, Rubin. *Healing Night: The Science and Spirit of Sleeping, Dreaming, and Awakening.* Minneapolis: Syren Book Company, 2006. Delicious must-read sleep book filled with science and sense.

Pinkola Estés, Clarissa. *Women Who Run With the Wolves: Myths and Stories of the Wild Woman Archetype.* New York: Ballantine Books, 1992. You'll soak up wisdom and reclaim your Wild Woman in every word.

ABOUT THE AUTHOR

Karen Brody is the founder of the Daring to Rest program for women. An expert in women's empowerment and well-being, with a passion for women's leadership, Karen helps women take back rest and dream big using yoga nidra meditation. Karen is certified in the Amrit Method of yoga nidra and trained in level two of iRest yoga nidra. She is also a writer and the playwright of *Birth*, a theater-for-social-change play seen in over seventy-five cities around the world. She has a BA in sociology from Vassar and an MA in women and international development from the International Institute of Social Studies in the Netherlands. She was raised in New York City and lives with her husband and two boys in Washington, DC.

For more, please visit Karen's website, daringtorest.com. There you can find Karen's blog, additional yoga nidra meditations, information about workshops, trainings, programs, and more.

ABOUT SOUNDS TRUE

Sounds True is a multimedia publisher whose mission is to inspire and support personal transformation and spiritual awakening. Founded in 1985 and located in Boulder, Colorado, we work with many of the leading spiritual teachers, thinkers, healers, and visionary artists of our time. We strive with every title to preserve the essential "living wisdom" of the author or artist. It is our goal to create products that not only provide information to a reader or listener, but that also embody the quality of a wisdom transmission.

For those seeking genuine transformation, Sounds True is your trusted partner. At SoundsTrue.com you will find a wealth of free resources to support your journey, including exclusive weekly audio interviews, free downloads, interactive learning tools, and other special savings on all our titles.

To learn more, please visit SoundsTrue.com/freegifts or call us toll-free at 800.333.9185.

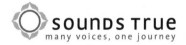